Following The Functional Path

Building and Rebuilding the Athlete

by **Vern Gambetta**

Cover Photos:
Soccer: Mark J. Rebilas/US PRESSWIRE
Football: Matt Cashore/US PRESSWIRE
Track and Field: Kirby Lee/US PRESSWIRE
Volleyball: CSPA/US PRESSWIRE
Swimming: Brian Spurlock/US PRESSWIRE

Cover Design and Typesetting: Trish Landsparger

Library of Congress Cataloging-in-Publication Data
Gambetta, Vern
        Following the Functional Path/Vern Gambetta
        ISBN 978-0-9842802-9-2
Copyright © by MomentumMedia Sports Publishing, Inc.
Printed in the United States of America

MomentumMedia Sports Publishing, Inc.
31 Dutch Mill Rd.
Ithaca, NY 14850
(607) 257-6970
info@MomentumMedia.com

Foreword

We live in a world where the information highway continues to grow at an astounding rate. Access to information is a key for us all as we negotiate each decision in our personal and professional lives. Unfortunately, within this information "super-highway," there is a lot of what I can only describe as "noise."

Un-truths, half-truths, spells, potions and marketing jargon clutter the ether and our education pathways. The blog is but one of the many vehicles available to us all as it allows for a short presentation of ideas and facts, sometimes unstructured and other times part of an overall plan or strategy. What is apparent from many blogs is the way that the fundamental principles of the author clearly come to light in the conversation.

My simple answer to this 21st century phenomenon of "noise" has been to trust in a few practitioners who have built their information on tried and tested experience over many years. In my 40 years of coaching I have had the pleasure of listening to and working with a number of practitioners who I would class as being masters. Vern Gambetta is one such practitioner. One of his greatest attributes is that he maintains consistency in his sharing of information. Sharing information has become one of those lost skills in recent times as more and more people think that there are secrets to improved performance. The truth, as explained by Vern, is that there are no secrets and that the process that leads to improved performance and reduced injury is a simple one.

As you explore Vern's thoughts and jottings it will become apparent that there is a clear link between life skills and experiences and sports skills and experiences. The two journeys are intertwined and he offers many examples of this interrelationship and how they impact our daily lives. You will also be encouraged to question your assumptions as he challenges thought across a range of issues. For some this may be stimulating and for others it may make you shout back with defiance—very healthy reactions in a world of apathy and "sleepwalking."

Enjoy Vern's words, thoughts and provocations.

Kelvin Giles

Veteran sport coach, world-renowned consultant, and founder and director of Movement Dynamics UK, Ltd., a company that provides athletic development services to all levels of athletes and sports organizations in Australia and throughout the world.

Introduction

This collection of writings is compiled from my blog posts from August 2005 through August 2010. I started writing my blog, Functional Path Training, as a daily writing "warm-up" exercise to get me focused on writing my book, *Athletic Development—The Art & Science of Functional Sports Conditioning*. It served me well. I finished the book late in the fall of 2005, but I kept writing because I found that it continued to give me a focus to start my day.

There are some consistent themes that run throughout the posts. A major theme is my ongoing fascination with innovation and change. As a pioneer in what is now called functional training I never thought that the work I was doing with my athletes was particularly innovative, but in others' eyes it was, and still is. You will gain insights into my thought process and the evolution of some training ideas. This is a continuing journey for me, hence the name, Following the Functional Path. The destination is performance in the competitive arena, but each new athlete and team represents a new excursion.

I write from a coach's perspective because that is what I am. I have been fortunate to coach at levels from middle school on up to the highest rankings of amateur and professional sport. As a coach I know how important it is to blend art and science. The two go hand in glove; you will see that theme reflected in the writings.

I am also a generalist whose approach to coaching is very eclectic. I have never been afraid to go outside sport for information and inspiration. To me that is part of traveling the functional path. I have always been willing to question—to probe beyond the what of training, to get to the why and how. I learned that if I knew the why, then I could reproduce the training method or technique in the context of my own system. I hope that these writings will give you some answers. If nothing else they may motivate you to ask more questions.

I do my best to recognize the many pioneers who blazed the functional path before me. The ideas and concepts collected here reflect the great mentors who have taught and motivated me. But ultimately it is the athletes who I have been privileged to work with— some famous and many anonymous—who, through their efforts, taught me about the wisdom of the body and how to train.

My hope is that this book will challenge and inspire you to venture out onto your own functional path. Enjoy the journey!

Vern Gambetta

You Can't Do That

Have you had people tell you that you could not do something? I have, and personally, I always took it as a challenge. Thank God I never listened to all the people who told me I could not do the things I have done. I truly believe people say this to put limits on others, because they cannot imagine doing the things they themselves say can't be done. I was labeled stupid more than once during my elementary and high school years, (I have the D's and F's to prove it), but somehow I have overcome my stupidity to write a few books. Don't ever take no for an answer. Don't let people tell you that you can't do something. Go out and do it, and prove them wrong. They told me we could never do the things in baseball that we did with the White Sox, but we did them and they worked. Everyone has been trying to imitate what we did ever since, with no idea why it worked. I could go on and on, but when I hear someone tell other people, especially a young person, that they can't do something, I get my dander up. Don't listen to the naysayers; go out and prove them wrong. That is what I try to do everyday.

Training Stuff: The Good, Bad & Ugly

I love training stuff. In fact I have boxes of videos of training stuff that I have collected over the years. I have shelves of books full of training stuff. Some of it is really cool looking and some of it is really dumb and ugly. Fortunately or unfortunately, I have tried much of this stuff. Some worked and some failed. I used to have to work really hard to find stuff. No longer. I can log onto YouTube or any one of thousands of exercise guru sites and find any kind of stuff that I want to see. But does this really put you or me ahead of the game? It is still just stuff. Is my stuff better than your stuff? How can we know?

I have given this much thought. I know the stuff that I have used has worked predictably well for the time that I have used it. Why do

I know it works? Very simply because 41 years ago when I started coaching, I realized that to get an edge as a coach and as an athlete I had to have a system. So I started working on putting my stuff into a context, a system. I tried to find out why some stuff worked and why some did not work. To do that I relied on scientific research and what we today call best practice. It was a constant prototyping process—trying stuff, fine tuning it, and trying it again. This is an ongoing process that I continue today. I am constantly working to upgrade the stuff, but always within the context of the sport and the athletes I am working with. So what's the point of this stuff about stuff? In order to make the stuff you do meaningful, get beyond the *what* stuff. Know and understand the *why,* and make sure you know the *how* and *when.* Then and only then will your stuff become meaningful and lead to positive training adaptations over time.

False Praise: A Slippery Slope

Good job. Well Done. If you go to any gym, practice field, pool or court around the world that is what you hear. I look at the action that was praised and say why? Was it really a good job? Was it really well done? No, sometimes it wasn't. Then why do we praise mediocre effort and outcomes? I think I know. It is because somewhere along the way we were told we needed to be positive, to raise self-esteem. Be honest. If it was a poor effort, point it out. You don't have to attack the person—that is not what it is about. It is the effort the person is giving. Praise and reward the effort—or conversely, criticize the effort. Just don't criticize the person. The athlete knows it is wrong and they begin to tune you out when you are constantly giving false praise. If you don't know what to say, don't say anything! Be real. You can help the athlete get better if you correct what needs to be corrected with a recommendation of something they can do to improve. That is how you raise self-esteem. You guide them toward their goal, praise exemplary effort and the outcome will follow.

I certainly believe in positive reinforcement and praise for great effort and outcomes. I also understand how important self-esteem and self-image are in teaching and coaching, but we have gone overboard with praise for mediocrity in order to build self-esteem. In every situation there are minimum expectations and standards that must be met to be part of the team. I emphasize minimum standards. Meeting those minimum standards does not warrant praise; those are expectations that everyone must meet. The same is true of effort. Everyone is expected to go all out, plain and simple, no exceptions. So to praise someone for going all out is hollow and meaningless.

We know from research and from results in front of our eyes everyday that false praise has the opposite effect. It makes the praise meaningless and ineffective, possibly even lowering self-esteem. Praise those efforts and actions that exceed expectations, not those that just meet expectations. If I see one more bumper sticker proclaiming their child an honor student, I am going to scream. Everyone can't be an honor student, everyone can't earn a varsity letter. There has to be a high standard to warrant an honor. Lets raise the bar, not lower it. The level of expectation definitely will determine the level of achievement. Praising average work as great trivializes great.

From a coach's perspective it seriously erodes your credibility and soon will render you ineffective. Be a John Wooden—select and measure your words carefully, instruct and teach, praise the extraordinary not the average. Hold yourself and those you teach and coach to a higher standard.

The Specificity Trap

As an athletic development coach you should beware of overdoing specificity—it can be a trap, a one-way dead-end street. You may be just adding stress to stress by too closely trying to overload the actual movements of the sport. You can get too specific and lose sight of what you are doing. My role as an athletic development coach is to prepare the athlete for the stress of their sport. I can do that in many ways without strictly trying to imitate the movements of the sport throughout training. They get enough of that in practice. There are times in a program to get very specific and other times to be very general. My basic litmus test is this: Are the movements that I use in training sport-appropriate? I look at it as a three-step process.

Step One— The sport itself is the domain of the sport coach, although they may enlist my help here.

Step Two—Stuff that looks like the sport, but is not the sport. I do some of this.

Step Three—Stuff that does not have any resemblance to the sport, but that will prepare the athlete for the demands of the sport. Distribute the work and the emphasis in training accordingly. It is simple and it seems to work.

Experience or Experiences

The older I get and the longer I teach and coach, the more I value learning from people who have had a multitude of experiences. One of my mentors, Joe Vigil, summed it up quite nicely for me 25 years ago. He said that there are many people who have 30 years of experience on their resume, but what they really have is one experience 30 times. I don't know about you, but I want to be around someone who has had a multitude of experiences—successes and failures, wins and losses. Those kinds of people are genuine; they are usually willing to share. Those are the people I want to learn from, not some over-confident know-it-all who has had one experience 30 times.

If you are just starting out in your career as a coach, look for someone who has fought the battles, who has had experiences, who has battle scars. Find a Yoda, not a poser or an imposter who has all the secrets. Call them up, go visit them, watch them coach and you will see the way and the light, so to speak. It is not about glitz and glamour; it is about being basic, honest, true to your beliefs, willing to risk and make mistakes and learn from them. I am so thankful for people like my former coaches, teachers and mentors. Bill Crow, the first coach I worked under who taught the value of organization and structure. Gene "Red" Estes who encouraged me to get into coaching. Sam Adams, who patiently coached me in the decathlon. Marshall Clark who gave me a chance to coach at Stanford and showed me the value of a steady even-tempered approach. Joe Vigil who still inspires me to keep learning, and countless others who helped me and shared what they know and did not know. I hope all of you who are in the formative stages of your career can find people like this to guide you and help you. Actually it does not matter where you are in your career, you always need people like this. I know I depend on the advice and counsel of many to help me in my coaching and teaching. I look for people who have substance, who are open and willing to share, who have no secrets and who are not seeking fame and fortune, to share and learn with.

Mental Toughness, Motivation and Teaching

One night, I was channel surfing and came upon a one-hour program on that year's preseason training of a

top 20-ranked football team. I usually don't watch this stuff, but I heard "mental toughness" so I decided to watch to see if I could learn what this was. I watched it and I'm still not sure what to think. I definitely did not learn what mental toughness was. It brought back some really bad memories of my college football days in the '60s. All the head coach and the other coaches talked about was mental toughness. Over and over they preached it. There was one coach who just screamed—no instruction, just screaming of mindless platitudes vaguely related to mental toughness. This left me cold. I have done my share of screaming, but over the years I learned that when I controlled my voice better the athletes responded and listened, and I was able to teach so much more. If you scream all the time they will tune you out. I have watched Jim Radcliffe (University of Oregon) with his players. He does not have to scream; he commands respect with his presence, his persona, his knowledge and his actions.

But this mental toughness thing bugs me. What is it? Everyone talks about it, but I have still not found a good explanation of it and how to teach it. Do mindless drills that elicit fatigue build it? Do punishment runs do it? Do trite slogans on the back of t-shirts enhance it? I just don't believe in it. I do, however, believe in mental discipline and athletic intelligence. Every great athlete I have seen has those qualities. Mental discipline is having your head in the practice, the training, and the game. It is being completely engaged and mindful. You show up everyday with a plan and a goal to help you execute the plan. You don't have to have someone screaming at you for motivation, because the leaders have set out the goals and the means to achieve those goals. You just need to put your nose to the grindstone and go after it.

Don't get me wrong, I am not some fluffy wimp who lets the athletes run the show. I believe that the coach is a teacher who must be firm and fair, must teach the athlete the qualities that make up mental discipline, and praise the efforts to achieve it. That does not mean you need to be any less demanding, you just need to lead and to teach. Leading and teaching will enhance mental disciple and increase athletic intelligence, both of which will give the athlete a chance to excel in the competitive arena.

The Basics: A Quick Review

First, let me start by saying that I had an amazing conversation recently with Jim Steen, the swim coach at Kenyon College. Under Jim's guidance the Kenyon men have won 31 straight Division III championships. For the first time in his career at Kenyon he will not be coaching the women, so that he can coach fewer people. We were talking about how he starts each season. He said that he starts each season with a clean slate; he starts out as if he knows nothing. Sure, better to start there than to think you have it figured out and you know everything. If there is a secret, this might be it.

He got me thinking, we should do the same with training—start with a clean slate, and assume you know nothing. The three movement constants are the most basic place to start. They are the body, gravity, and the ground. Every time you begin a new training program this is where you must start. Training is how these constants interact to achieve optimum results.

The body is what we are trying to improve. The body is a self-organizing organism that will respond to the stress placed upon it in training. If the training is adequate, then it will respond positively. If it is too easy, there will be minimal adaptive response. If it is too hard, it will shut down. Adaptation takes time and it is cumulative over time.

Gravity is always there. We live in a gravitationally enriched environment. Gravity loads us. We are in a constant struggle with gravity. Strength training enhances our ability to work with and against gravity. Gravity will always win, and although we may be able to cheat it at certain times and in certain situations, it will prevail.

The ground is where we live, work and play. The ability to use the ground effectively to produce force is crucial to training adaptation in terms of force production, force reduction, speed, and movement enhancement.

I know this seems simple and it is, but it is not simplistic. It does not take much to mix and match the constants to the demands of the sport and to end with a quite complex program. Complexity is not the goal; it is a logical outcome of working on the three movement constants.

The Body as a Machine

The mechanistic view of the body is passé. The body is not a machine. You can't turn muscles on and off, and there are no switches to activate or deactivate muscles or, for that matter, energy systems. I struggle to understand what is going on when I hear statements like, "The glute is not firing" or "I need to activate that muscle." These statements demean the wisdom of the body; the body is so much smarter than that.

Muscles do not turn on and off; they are always on. Within one movement a muscle can perform many different functions, depending on the requirements of the task (the movement problem that is being solved). Muscles do not work in isolation. They in work in synergy with other muscles to produce smooth, efficient movement. When there is a problem with the movement, there is usually a problem of coordination between muscle groups.

I think the misunderstanding arises because of the way we are taught traditional anatomy, which focuses on individual muscles and how they are innervated. It is a mentally convenient approach that does not reflect the realities of movement. We do not move and function in the anatomical position. The body is designed to solve movement problems. As coaches, teachers and therapists we need to present the body with increasingly complex problems to solve. Different individuals find different solutions to the same problem. That is okay. That is what makes the body special. If we all did everything the same way we would be robots and all we would have to do is reprogram ourselves and replace parts. Frankly, as a coach that does not appeal to me. I love the variability and the challenge of helping guide the athlete toward solutions to their movement problems. It is a constant challenge that resists a formulaic approach. I must use sound principles and apply them individually. I urge you to embrace the challenge.

Training Basics

Keep it basic. The complexity will come by combining basic elements. Be targeted and focused. Never lose sight of the goal: to prepare the athlete to be taken to their physical, technical and psychological limits in the competitive arena. Training is a means to an end—nothing more, nothing less. Constantly apply the following litmus test to your training: Is what I am doing *nice-to-do* or *need-to-do*? If it is not *need-to-do*, don't do it. From my experience, nice-to-do activities make you tired and hurt; *need-to-do* makes you better and helps you advance toward your training and competition goals.

Some Thoughts on Recovery

I remember returning from my first trip to Australia totally enthralled with what I had seen in terms of systematic recovery programs at the AIS (Australian Institute of Sport) and some of the state institutes. I came to the conclusion at the time that you must be proactive and design your training around recovery. Conceptually that might have been a logical conclusion especially with the attitude that existed here in the States at the time. That attitude was that rest and recovery were a luxury. You rested when you needed it—a very reactive attitude.

Over the last 14 years I have seen the whole "recovery" piece take on a life of its own. It seems an elite athlete cannot do more that a few minutes of "hard" training and they must have a massage, get ice and have a specially concocted recovery drink. In other words, the pendulum has swung completely to the other side where it seems to be all about recovery and not about training.

The truth lies somewhere in between. The human body is a wonderfully adaptive and self-organizing organism. We need to give it credit and stop interfering with the natural inflammatory cascade that triggers the adaptive response. I think we need to take a step back and look at what we are doing with recovery today and reassess its place in the whole training process.

There is very little actual research to back up what we are doing in recovery. Let's reconsider how often and what external means of recovery we are using. Let's do a better job of learning what each athlete's "recoverability" is in relation to all the various types of work they use in training. Let's remember that the foundation for a good training program is a good plan. A good plan will take into account the demands of the various types of work and adjust accordingly. Hopefully this will stimulate some thought and discussion and we will find a more balanced approach to recovery.

The Tyranny of Dead Ideas

Do you ever wonder why we keep teaching and following certain things, never questioning them? This tyranny of dead ideas stifles innovation and holds us back. It seems generation after generation falls prey to this and keeps repeating the mistakes of the previous generation. Imitation is not innovation. We have to be willing to let go of cherished beliefs that do not work, and in many cases are counterproductive. Here are a few that I see day-to-day in my work:

1. Necessity of an aerobic base for anaerobic exercise, start/stop, intermittent sprint, and transition game sports.
2. Icing a healthy limb after exercise.
3. The traditional model of periodization—volume to intensity, with a long period of general preparation to build a base.
4. The use of the down sweep pass in the 400-meter relay.
5. Jogging to warm up.
6. Static stretch to warm up.
7. Training to failure.

There are many more. Ask why. Is there a better way? Instead of blindly following ideas, question. Base your questioning on principles, not fads. Be willing to forge a new path and find better ways.

Keep It Simple and You Are Brilliant

How many times have we heard coaches evoke the KISS (Keep It Simple, Stupid) principle? When I hear KISS I almost take it as an insult, because it smacks of a dumbing down. I have believed for years that simplicity yields complexity. Start simple and basic and build complexity as needed. If it is not needed then don't go to more complexity. Simple is not necessarily simplistic.

I also strongly believe that if I can't explain the science to my athletes in terms that they can understand, then I probably should not be doing it. Why? Because if I can't explain it then I probably don't understand it, and if I don't understand it then it is not worth doing because it is going to be half-baked. It is just monkey-see monkey-do activities. I have found that the most brilliant people I know can make abstract concepts totally comprehensible, which is a gift of great teachers and coaches. I end with a quote from Winnie-the-Pooh: "It's more fun to talk to someone who doesn't use long difficult words, but rather short easy words like, 'What about lunch?'"

The Edge

I know many of you are seeking the edge in training. For many years I was doing the same. I was searching for secrets— the latest and the greatest, something special, that 1 or 2 percent that would make the difference. The more I searched the more elusive it became. Finally, I realized I had the answer right in front of me, but I could not see the forest for the trees. I had seen it time and again and missed it. In fact, I had done it and rejected it several times as unsophisticated, too simple.

So what is the edge? It is mindful, deliberate practice that never strays from the foundations of physical literacy and the fundamentals of the sport. The problem is that to constantly stress fundamentals seems mundane. It is the fundamentals that make the difference between staying injury free and getting injured. It is the fundamentals that are the foundation; the fundamentals must be constantly reinforced. I find that as a coach I must coach the fundamentals daily, just like the outstanding coaches who I have seen do the same. I now feel with a high degree of certainty that the search for the 2 percent is almost an exercise in futility. That final 2 percent will come if you take care of the first 98 percent. This is not to imply that you should stop learning and experimenting. By all means, keep learning and refining in order to keep the edge razor sharp. It takes time and correct timing of the application of all the elements of training. Take another look at your training. Stop looking for an edge and coach the basics. You will be surprised at the results.

The Planning Process

I am not saying this is the only way, but it is a method that works for me in my system. It is definitely more qualitative than quantative. We won the regional championship and finished fourth in the state championship.

I thought this would be helpful to you if I shared the process I use to begin a new training program. It is a blend of art and science with a heavy dose of experience thrown in. It is important to remember that this is the beginning of the third year of working with this team. The rising seniors and a couple of the juniors are at a relatively advanced training age and have an excellent work capacity. This will enable me to do some advanced work with them. This will be the first year we will have access to the weight room, whereas for the past two years we trained in the parking lot. I have mixed feelings about this. The parking lot made us tougher, as we had to improvise and endure the elements. I am concerned about distractions in the weight room. I will evaluate this immediately and adjust accordingly.

Steps in Designing a Training Program
Venice Volleyball Training Program for 2009

Step 1: Meet with head coach
Review last season
Competition results and schedule
Review training
Evaluate individual players (subjective)
Go over potential position changes in '09
Determine goals (training emphasis for '09)
Individualize more
Significantly improve jumping
(both approach and block)
Improve hitting power (arm speed)
Emphasize "quick speed" (court coverage)
More explosive power

Determine athletic development themes
    One step at a time or faster, higher, stronger.
    We will discuss with the team and get their input.
    I will develop a performance handbook that each
    player will receive in the spring. It will detail goals
    and workouts.

**Step 2: Review sport demands and any rule changes
that could affect style of play.**
This may seem obvious but I never take anything for
granted. If nothing else, this keeps me on target.

**Step 3: Review sports science and training literature
for anything new.**
I want to make sure that any techniques we are teaching
reflect the most current research.

Step 4: Look at club and school schedule for '09
This is still being finalized but I know when districts and
state playoffs are so that I can plan back from there.

Step 5: Classify competitions
Developmental
Important
Crucial
This will not be done until the summer or when the
school schedule is completed.

Step 6: Determine key dates
    Spring break (two training days—one with me and one
    with captains.)
    Midterms and finals (back off significantly here.)
    Auburn team camp

Step 7: Evaluate last year's training
    Number of days—essentially this went as planned, really
    nailed it in-season.

Content—needs improvement. Need to do better job of grouping the players.

In January, we will train Monday, Tuesday and Thursday. In February, we will add another session on Wednesday.

In the spring, club workouts are Sunday afternoons, Tuesday and Wednesday nights.

Step 8: Determine testing and need for testing

I will not do the amount of testing that I would like. This is simply due to the fact that I cannot be there all the time and I have no one to help me. Therefore, I have to use training as testing. We do some sort of balance single leg squat work daily in warm-up, so that is daily diagnostic. I use their progress in single-leg squat and their ability to handle the progression as feedback as to their training progress. I want to video more and use Dartfish, but once again it is a matter of time.

Step 9: The Plan

BLOCK ONE—Foundation (January 12 – February 28)
Theme: Re-establish the Base and Routine of Training

BLOCK TWO—Basic I (March 2 – April 10)
Theme: Get Strong

BLOCK THREE—Basic II (April 13 – May 15)
Theme: Get Fast

BLOCK FOUR—Build-up I (May 18 – June 26)
Theme: Power Up

BLOCK FIVE—Build-up II (June 29 –July 18)
Theme: Tune Up

BLOCK SIX—Pre-Competition (July 20 – August 7)
Theme: Get Functionally Fit

BLOCK SEVEN—Pre-season (August 10 – August 30)
Theme: Get Specific

BLOCK EIGHT—Early Competition (August 31 – October 11)
Theme: Sharpen and Focus

BLOCK NINE—Late Competition (October 12 – November 1)
Theme: Recharge the Battery and Fine Tune

BLOCK TEN— Peak Competition
(November 2 – November 21)
Theme: Go For the Gold!

Clueless in Sarasota

When is it good to be clueless? Maybe being oblivious is a better option. The more I see on the Internet, and read unedited, unreviewed stuff, the more I think it is good to be a bit clueless. If being clued in means cluttering my brain with a plethora of mindless information that focuses on the trivialization of training, then I prefer to be clueless. How can anyone filter the massive volume of information that is being produced by the day, hour and minute? You cannot, unless you have a context for your search for knowledge.

Context is king. You must have a historical context and a knowledge base in classical training and sport science literature as a firm foundation. I choose to remain clueless in my little world by expanding my knowledge with a plan and a direction. I had someone ask me if I read a certain blog or subscribed to a certain pay-for-play site. My answer was quite direct and succinct: I'm not interested in infomercials and the promotion of a new DVD.

Same with some of the debates I see: Does it really matter if it is inner core or outer core? Let's get real. At age 63 and after 41 years of coaching I am more motivated to learn than at anytime in my life, but I know I must separate the noise from the music, the wheat from the chaff. I am confident in what I do know and equally confident in what I do not know. My mind, my eyes and my ears are open. There are only so many bytes free so I want to focus on quality and the information I need to know to improve my knowledge. I choose to remain clueless with a childlike curiosity in my pursuit of excellence.

General Strength—A Closer Look

General strength (GS) has become a meaningless, throw-away term in the track and field world. You can give the circuits all kinds of cute names like Waterloo, Dunkirk or D-Day, but whatever name you use, they have evolved into mindless repetition of poor quality movements with no specific goal in mind. I remind you that just getting someone tired is not training with a purpose—it is just getting someone tired. Hurdle overs and unders are great if they're placed in the correct place in a workout; if not, they are just stuff.

If you look at the composition of the various GS workouts proliferating on many Internet sites, what you see is too much work in prone and supine positions with no discernible pattern or sequence to the movements. In a recent experience with a group of elite middle distance and distance runners, I observed this first hand. I could see no sequence to the application of the circuits and the distribution of the work throughout the training cycles. I was uncomfortable with it then and I am more uncomfortable now that it has taken on a life of its own. With middle distance and distance runners this has replaced strength training with appropriate resistance. What everyone calls GS (general strength) is really circuit training. It has a place in a program, but you must develop strength before you can endure it. The guiding principle is to develop strength before strength endurance, and power before power endurance.

Circuit training can and should be used during certain phases of the training year to enhance strength endurance and/or power endurance, depending on the composition of the circuit and the work-to-rest ratios and resistance. The movements need to be carefully chosen to fit the athlete's event, their specific needs and the time of the training year. I encourage you to take a long, hard look at how you are using this component. If it is just stuff thrown together, then it is just stuff. Anyone can do stuff.

Thoughts on Middle Distance and Distance Training

Here are some of my thoughts on training middle distance and distance runners. I continue to be amazed at the things that I see going on in training. We have been down this path so many times before that I am amazed that the same questions are being asked and the same mistakes are repeated. In my 41-year coaching career I have been fortunate to work with some great middle distance and distance athletes (male and female) and some great coaches. Here are some of the things I have learned.

> *Anyone can run miles.* It is what you put into the miles that count. More miles can make you tired, but they do not necessarily make you better.

> *Stop slogging.* Slow running and shuffling are poor foot strikes that just reinforce poor biomechanics.

> *Work on race distribution not race pace.* Races are never run at even pace. Learn to change gears. Learn your race and how you best need to run that race, and train accordingly.

> *Become race "hardened."* Learn how to race. The only way you can learn how to race is to race. Race over your race distance

and under your race distance. If you are an 800- or 1500-meter runner, try to run the second or third leg in a 4 x 400 relay as much as possible.

Always include an element of speed in training at all times of the year. If you are waiting to start speed work you are waiting to get beat.

Running strength comes from an accumulation of training over time.

Progress in your volume by adding training sessions, not by adding more to a session. If you are running once a day, add two morning sessions a week. If you are running five days a week, add a day. Progress gradually; never compromise good mechanics or quality.

Strength training must be an integral part of the runner's preparation during all phases of the year. You must train leg strength. Strength is the basis for speed and injury prevention. A good, comprehensive functional strength training program will help with postural integrity, joint integrity and shock absorption.

Use Bowerman's axiom of a hard day followed by an easy day. Make hard/easy your mantra.

Read Run, Run, Run *by Fred Wilt and* Modern Training for Running *by Ken Doherty.* Both were written more than 40 years ago. I know you will think I am living in the past, but both these books are spot-on with clear messages and information that today's coaches need. They are not confused by scientific gobbledygook, just good coaching information.

Some Powerful Thoughts

The first thought is for pushy eager parents and coaches who want to identify the "champion" early and dictate every move to the youngster. In the June 28, 2010 edition of *The New Yorker*, Calvin Tomkins wrote an article titled, "Anxiety on the Grass," in which he quotes Roger Federer's mother:

> *Roger had unbelievable coordination at a very young age. At age one he could kick a soccer ball in your direction. We noticed this but we didn't push him. All the major decisions of his sports career he took himself.*

Give them the space and they will grow.

The second thought is for coaches and teachers. It is from an article written by Lee Jenkins for the June 28, 2010 issue of *Sports Illustrated* titled, "Dynasty: Beginning or Ending?" about Phil Jackson, coach of the Lakers:

> *What separates Jackson are the speeches he doesn't give, the timeouts he doesn't call, the spaces he forces his players to fill on their own. "It's like going to a psychologist," says former Bulls center Will Perdue. "He doesn't give you the answers. He expects you to figure it out for yourself."*

White space on a page and silence can send a stronger message than loud speech.

Game Speed

This was at the forefront of my mind when I watched the World Cup matches. Game speed is different than pure track speed. Game speed requires the player to quickly—instantly—solve

a myriad of movement problems. The track sprinter has one task—
get to the finish line as fast as possible. The sprinter deals with three
dimensions: the body, gravity, and the ground. The games player has
a fourth, and some would say, a fifth dimension—the opposition as
well as an implement (like a racket, and/or a ball).

The sprinter is rewarded for time in the air—the time necessary to
recover the legs in the stride cycle. The games player is penalized
for time in the air—the requirements of triple extension to start and
accelerate and triple flexion to stop, demand that the feet are close
to the ground. Also, there is a demand for highly variable stride
lengths and frequencies. Therefore, stride frequency is rewarded.
Game speed is totally dynamic and unpredictable, and in many ways
random and chaotic.

Are sprint speed and game speed related? Yes, absolutely. They are
cousins. The research of Warren Young from the University of Ballarat
in Australia shows that the more complex the cuts and changes of
direction, the less correlation with linear sprint speed. I prefer to
have good sprint speed as a basis to teach and develop game speed.
Obviously a combination of the two gives that player an edge,
provided he or she can channel that sprint speed to the demands of
the game.

Game speed entails the ability to recognize, react, start, accelerate,
decelerate, possibly reaccelerate and change direction, and stop
quickly. Quickly is a time from tenths-of-a-second to four to seven
seconds depending on the game or situation in the game. To
improve game speed you must know the speed demands of the
game you are preparing for, the player's position, and the player's
speed, strength and power qualities. I have found it most important
to understand how each player plays their game and help them to
improve that. Generic cone, ladder, ring, and programmed change
of direction drills have varying degrees of transfer to improve game
speed. Overall we probably spend too much time on these types of
drills.

Training for game speed demands intensity and focused concentration applied to quality repetitions. There is a tendency to introduce fatigue too early in the process. Mindless repetition of drills has been proven to be ineffective. Remember, just making them tired is not making them better. Teach first, refine the movements, then speed it up. Only then should you add an element of fatigue.

Another axiom that I live by is that testing speed does not equal game speed. Testing speed typically involves programmed and rehearsed situations; the game is unrehearsed and random. Game speed is hard to measure unless you have sophisticated analysis systems to use. If you do, then the job becomes a bit easier and more specific. If not, you must closely observe practice, study videos of practice and game situations, and adjust and train accordingly.

It is important to always try to incorporate speed of thought, decision-making and awareness in game speed training. That is fundamental to insuring a degree of transfer of training to the game. Game speed training should consist of short, sharp bouts of work with a specific goal for the movement that the player clearly understands. At various times it is valuable to slow it down in order to speed it up. The next step is chaining those bouts together in varying sequences and actions. Then add a reaction component, and last but not least, add an opponent or a ball.

Training game speed is a challenging process. It demands thorough preparation by the coach to constantly assess progress and challenge the athlete. Be creative—it is a *FUNdamental* challenge.

Should We Listen to You?

A post by noted author and blogger Seth Godin, on June 26, 2010, struck home with me. I have been thinking lately about paying your dues and how you earn the right to be heard. In today's world anyone can get on the Internet and start making noise. Someone will listen to the noise and pass it on. The person who generates the most noise is now considered an *expert*. The problem is that there is no substance, but now they are an expert. Just like you can't enlist in the army as a General, I think you have to pay your dues and earn the right to be heard. Here are Seth Godin's criteria for earning the right to being heard:

- Be informed.
- Be rational.
- Pay your dues.
- Have a platform where a lot of people can hear you.
- Be an impacted constituent, not a gadfly.
- Represent a tribe of people with similar concerns.
- You've been right before.
- You're not anonymous.
- You have a previous relationship and permission to interrupt.
- Listening to you earns something of value.

Paying your dues is a process, and in many a journey. You gain experiences, learn from your mistakes, take risks, and constantly challenge yourself and those you work with to learn and to improve.

Change and Innovation

Change is a constant. We are not the same now as we were minutes, or even seconds, ago. On a macro level, change—and its partner, innovation—can be uncomfortable. It is very easy to say you must embrace change, but then actually doing it is another thing. I have found that change for the sake of change ultimately does nothing. I think if we change with a purpose, then change can be lasting and meaningful.

Innovation and change are closely related. To innovate you have to learn to see the world with new eyes. You have to think like a child, wipe away all those preconceived notions, and have a clean slate. So many people who claim to be innovators are really imitators. Imitation is not innovation. To quote my colleague Kelvin Giles, a coach for 40-plus years, "Coaches are change engineers." We must find ways to problem solve and lead change or we will not produce results with our athletes. To innovate you need to plant the seeds of innovation through deep practice, continual learning, and skill enhancement. Start with the basics. You can't write the great American novel if you don't know the alphabet. To paraphrase Gandhi, be the change you want to see.

Getting Strong: The Mode and Method

Sometimes we get too wrapped up in the mode of strength training and lose sight of what we are trying to accomplish. Select a mode of strength training that is appropriate to the sport you are training for. Do not lock yourself into one mode. For example, pulling movements can be accomplished in a variety of ways using a variety of implements. It all depends on the ultimate goal. If you accept that strength training is a means to an end, not an end unto itself, a whole new vista of options becomes available. I just keep reminding myself that strength training is coordination training with appropriate resistance. The key words here are coordination training and appropriate resistance. I do not get as hung up on chasing numbers as I once did. I know there are certain landmarks that the athlete must achieve based on gender, training age, skill level, and sport and I let those guide me. I do not try to get crazy selecting the mode. Start with body weight and go to weight vests, sandbags, dumbbells and bars. The other rule I live by is nice-to-do/have versus need-to-do/have. Use common sense, be basic and fundamental, and you can build strength that you can use and apply in your sport.

Getting Strong: Preparation

Getting strong is relatively easy, but preparing to get strong is hard. This is not to demean or disparage anyone's ideas, rather it is a reaction to what I have seen throughout my career. It is easy to get someone on a strength training program and load them up and make very significant measurable strength gains on traditional exercises in relatively short periods of time. There is nothing wrong with traditional exercises—we need them and they have a place. What I have seen, though, is a lack of an investment in preparation to get strong. This previously came from traditional physical education, which included a myriad of movement skills that emphasized the ability to handle body weight in many different positions and angles. To prepare to get strong demands starting with the ability to handle body weight exercises and building across a continuum progressing to the heavy external loading appropriate for the sport or activity you are training for. It is a process—slow and methodical in most cases.

With postpubertal boys who have a huge anabolic advantage, the temptation is to load them quickly. Even though they respond, this is a mistake. Taking a year or longer to carefully and methodically progress, learn and master correct technique will result in significantly greater strength gains in the long term. In addition it will serve to protect the athlete from injury. I like to think of it as an investment in long-term strength gain. Build structural strength, great joint integrity, and sound technique but also be sure to develop other athletic qualities in parallel to the strength development. This is not revolutionary; it is common sense. Give a little at the beginning and get a lot at the end.

Ultimately, we have to get them strong and to do that you need external resistance. If the sport demands that you move another person or propel a heavy object, then those demands are different than if you are preparing to hit a golf ball. The girls on my volleyball team who have gone through the progression were all able to squat one-and-a-half times their body weight. Is that necessary to be a great volleyball player? I am not sure, but one thing I do know is that their ability to handle jumping loads has increased significantly. In some cases it took three years to get to that level; in another, one year. It really depends on the adaptability and trainability of the athlete. In summary, to get them strong, invest in the preparation necessary to get them strong.

Fit for What?

I just watched a video of a team training for the World Cup. Frankly it looked like track practice. The question you must ask is: What are you getting fit for? Are you getting fit for a six-minute run test or for the match? You must run with a purpose. Running willy-nilly around the pitch is not rewarded. Soccer is basically a big physical chess game where creating and exploiting space is rewarded. That requires more than just being able to run forever. Johan Cruyff, Dutch star from the '70s and later a very successful coach, put it quite well in a June 2, 2010 *New York Times* article titled "How a Soccer Star is Made," by Michael Sokolove: "Don't run so much; you have to be in the right place at the right moment, not too early, not too late." The message is simple: Train for the match—not what you think is occurring, but what is actually happening.

Skill Training:
Quantum versus Newtonian View

The Newtonian view of skill training is to construct neat little training packages that are programmed to proceed logically step-by-step in a linear manner to a higher degree of proficiency. Don't get me wrong. There is a place for this, but much less than we once thought. Too much of this creates robots who look good until the competition starts. You must have skill and drill progressions, but they must be criteria-based so that every athlete is not asked to progress at the same rate. Each athlete has a very distinct movement fingerprint. No two athletes in the same sport or event move exactly alike.

A quantum, and definitely more contemporary, view of this is to present the athlete with a series of increasingly difficult and different movement problems to solve. To do that, we must give them the tools to solve those problems by providing a good foundation of basic movement skill, strength to control their bodies, and some knowledge of the end goal. We know, based on volumes of current neuroscience research, that the brain and the nervous system are very plastic, self-organizing and highly adaptable. Together, they are not a computer; that analogy does not give the nervous system the credit it deserves. Ten thousand hours is a number tossed around now, but it is not just putting in mindless repetition for ten thousand hours. It is an accumulation of experiences through mindful, meaningful, deep practice. There is success and failure—you learn from both and self-correct. Look closely at what you are doing. Create a rich and varied learning environment. You must encourage experimentation and risk-taking to keep expanding the performance envelope. I encourage you to think beyond programmed drills and get creative to help your athletes' ability to solve complex movement problems.

Sport Appropriate Training

What do I mean by sport-appropriate training? I use the term sport-appropriate training to differentiate from sport-specific training. Sport specific is the actual movement of the sport. In swimming, it would be swimming a specific stroke; in basketball it would be shooting, dribbling, passing and defending. It is practice of the sport.

Sport appropriate would consist of training methods and activities that are similar but not the same. Working on component movements—for example, running or swimming with resistance. Bounding for a sprinter would be appropriate during certain phases of the year, but not specific, because of the longer ground contact time. The distinction is sometimes fine, but I think it is important. I do think that sometimes we get caught up in trying to imitate the movements of the sport and then those imitations have very little direct transfer. I always want to be efficient with my training; I want the highest degree of transfer possible. I have found that using the sport-appropriate concept as a filter has helped me have a better focus in my training. Once again, I prefer to spend time on the *need-to-do* rather that just kill time with the *nice-to-do*.

Advice: Just Do YOUR Job

Something I am observing more and more is people wanting to be something they are not. Start with the coach. The coach wants to be a therapist or a scientist. The ATC (Certified Athletic Trainer) wants to be a physical therapist. The physical therapist wants to be an MD. The MD . . . well, not sure on that. In many cases they want to be entrepreneurs and some are coaching wannabes. The sport scientist wants to be a coach without being accountable for the results in competition, unless they are spectacular and they can claim success. Parents definitely want to be coaches. Here is a simple solution: Everyone do your job and do it well. Know enough about what everyone else does so that you can communicate with the other professionals, parents, and boosters, but do your job. Know what you know and what you don't know, and do the best with what you have.

Voice Crying Out in the Dark: Where Are the Coaches?

I feel like a voice crying out in the dark again. I have never been one to hold my thoughts in, so here goes. Where have all the coaches gone? I see a plethora of exercise science, human movement science, sport science, and kinesiology graduates, but where are the coaches? No one wants to sweat; no one wants to get dirty and rake the long jump pit. I am definitely not anti-sport science; I think my record speaks for itself in that regard. But who is training coaches? What happened to the good old-fashioned coaching methods classes taught by coaches who were coaching? I really don't care if you can diagram the Krebs cycle forward and backward, or any other scientific minutiae. Can you teach? Can you coach? Can you demonstrate the activity you are teaching? We need to get way back to basics here.

When I watch sports at every level I see poor coaching running rampant—poor basic movement fundamentals, poor sport skills, poor practice organization, and on and on. A huge reason why is that we no longer have coaches who are trained as teachers. They don't know how to teach, because they were never taught how to teach. You should never criticize without offering a solution. Unfortunately, the solutions are somewhat expensive and complex. With all the cutbacks in education it would be tough to require coaches to be trained. Right now in many sports, schools and clubs will take anyone they can get for low wages or for free. It is going to take time to rectify this situation. Certainly the USOC (United States Olympic Committee) and the various sport governing bodies could play a much more active role, but I am not sure they recognize the problem. You can't go to the cause of the problem for a solution. We need to educate the end user—the athletes and the parents—to know what constitutes good coaching. We need to emphasize that coaching is teaching and that you can learn to be a better coach.

Last but not least, we need to emphasize that the measure of a good coach is not wins, but the quality of teaching and the experience the coach provides for the athlete.

Never Too Old

I recently spoke at length to one of my coaching heroes and mentors, Nort Thornton, former men's swimming coach at the University of California, Berkeley. Now a volunteer assistant, Nort is in his late 70s, with certainly nothing left to prove. He has coached world record holders and Olympic champions. He has done it all, but is still curious and trying to improve himself. He is never satisfied that he has the answer.

He had a couple of the books that I had recommended to him and we discussed some of the ideas in them. Then, he proceeded to share with me an idea that he had regarding putting more pressure on the little finger in the swim stroke. He got the idea from a book he had read about strength training. I listened in astonishment and awe. I was thinking, who else is thinking about pressure on the little finger to help better engage the lats? I went home, dove in the pool and fooled with it a bit. Certainly intriguing, but you know it is really not about the idea; it is about the man. People like Nort inspire and challenge me. He is everything a coach should be, and still going everyday after 60-plus years of coaching. Today, when you go out to work with your athletes, regardless of the sport, think of Nort. Look at the athletes and the sport you are working with differently. How can you get better, to make the athletes better? Challenge yourself like he challenges himself. I wish there were more Nort Thorntons in coaching.

Strength Training Fundamentals

Strength training in a seven-day training cycle must include pulling movements, pushing movements,

squat and squat derivative movements, rotational movements and bracing movements. Pick the specific exercises appropriate to your sports and training age. Once again simplicity yields complexity. Don't try to make it complicated.

Focus on the Workout

In many ways just writing a workout is quite easy, especially with the ability to easily cut and paste. Just go to last year's workouts at the same phase, copy and paste, make a few adjustments and you are good to go. If it is just about the workout, then I guess that is fine, but the workout is so much more than sets and reps, distances and intervals. The workout is the essential building block of the whole training plan. Each workout is a step toward the ultimate competitive goal.

This year is not the same as last year—a different group, a year older in chronological age and some more than a year older in training age. I probably spend 30 minutes a day planning the details of each training session—more time if you consider the thinking time before the pen hits the paper. Each workout should have a specific measurable or observable objective. The athletes need to know what that objective is, as this is their target for the day. The workout must meet the objectives of the training phase and be in context of the workout that preceded it and those to follow. Then there is the individual in the group context. I must make sure to communicate what each individual needs to do, and sometimes this is more a management issue than one of training methodology.

When my volleyball team is in the middle of finals, I want to make sure that that we stabilize the gains we have made, get them focused for about 30 to 35 minutes, and get them back to studying. Simply said, but more difficult to achieve. First, I need to get their attention and get them focused on the task at hand, not tomorrow's exam. That really starts before the workout by engaging each athlete in a short conversation about school, the weekend, and then what she needs to do today. When the workout is finished, objectively evaluate the workout in the context of the whole plan and today's objectives. Use that evaluation to begin the process of planning for the next session. Remember, a long-term training plan is a collection of individual workouts building toward a specific goal.

Sport Science is Good, But...

I just finished reading an outstanding coaching book: *Four Champions, One Gold Medal: The true story of four swimmers who battled for the same Olympic dream*, by Chuck Warner (1999). It has some real insights into what it takes to compete and win at the highest level. You definitely have to get comfortable with being uncomfortable all the time. This book has some great insights if you read between the lines. Even if you don't, this is a great chronicle of a different era.

This section struck me as particularly relevant to what I see as a move away from coaching to more sport science:

During the 1980s many American coaches sought more effective training methods through better utilization of scientific testing. Unfortunately, many scientists attempted to provide coaches with new, scientifically-based training methodologies rather than study existing programs, learn why they were successful and help coaches improve them. For many well-intentioned coaches and scientists, this created what Thomas Huxley once called, "The tragedy of a single fact killing a theory." Training programs that were proven from experience, and developed on the basis of a coach's theory, were often discarded in favor of a program based on a few, or even a single, isolated fact.

Although science has a great deal to contribute to the success of all athletes, including distance swimmers, it must be filtered through the mind of a coach's theory based on experience. Anyone who has been a swimming coach for five or ten years should be able to begin to draw his own conclusions from science, research and other coaches' training programs.

No sport scientist ever invented a viable technique or training method. As coaches we must work with the sport scientist and understand sport science, but ultimately we must coach. Three of the four swimmers' programs detailed in this book are coach driven and athlete centered, which is the road to success.

More Lessons Learned

1. Define yourself.
2. Know what you don't know.
3. Know what you do know.
4. Beware of false prophets bearing gifts.
5. Have a good working compass oriented to true north.
6. Coaching is about people and relationships not x's and o's.
7. Those who scream and yell the loudest don't get heard.
8. Doing the grunt work enables you to make the fun stuff even more fun.
9. Never compromise your core principles or beliefs.
10. Friendship is one of the most valuable things you can have.
11. True friends are there in the good times and the bad.
12. Honor and respect those who have opened the door and blazed the path for you.
13. Family first!
14. Quick fixes and crash programs don't work.
15. There are no secrets.

Then and Now—Were the Good Old Days Really So Good?

I have seen and heard much discussion regarding how different kids are today. I hear that they are lazy, unfit, disrespectful and they just won't do the things that kids did 40 or 50 years ago. Since I am still involved in the day-to-day coaching of high school athletes I have also given this issue much thought. I guess the perspective of coaching 41 years at all levels of competition gives me some insights that others who started later may not have. I also have been a classroom teacher in history and geography, a teacher of physical education and a coach of multiple sports.

Two preparatory points are necessary:

1. The older you get, the easier it is to remember the good of the "good old days" and forget the bad.
2. We live in an entirely different world today than 41 years ago.

Those points being made, please indulge me as I attempt to explain what I see in kids today.

Let's look at *then* first:
- Students rode bikes or walked to school.
- Kids had mandatory daily physical education.
- Most kids started playing three sports in elementary or middle school and then narrowed it down to two by high school.
- Family structure was still there.
- You seldom saw a latchkey kid.
- Less litigation.
- No high fructose corn syrup.
- No professionalization of youth and high school sports.
- Sports were centered in the schools and recreation departments.

- Parents were interested, but not directly involved.
- There were virtually no competitive opportunities for girls.
- Coaches were usually trained teachers, often physical education teachers.
- Coaches were the experts, because in many cases they were.
- Coaches did not specialize, they coached multiple sports.
- A sporting event on TV was special because there was were not many of them.
- No national high school or youth championships.
- No shoe contract—you wore Converse or Keds, and black or white was the choice of colors.
- There were strict transfer rules—no changing schools in midyear because you did not like the coach or you were not starting.

Let's look at *now*:
- Students drive or ride in cars to school.
- No mandatory physical education and little or no recess.
- Kids specialize in one sport from an early age.
- Sports are centered outside the schools.
- Coaches are not trained as educators; in essence, anyone can be a coach.
- Parents are involved; they run and have ownership of school and club programs because of fundraising.
- National championships in youth sports and high school sports.
- Sports are on television 24/7.
- Our diet is worse than most Third World nations.
- Kids spend hours a day on computers and cell phones.
- The only time many kids play is at an organized practice.
- We have more knowledge in sports medicine and sport science.
- We have significantly better facilities.
- Unlimited competitive opportunities for boys and girls.
- If you are not a starter or a star you either quit or transfer.

So what is the conclusion? First of all, you cannot separate sport from society. I have always felt sport is a reflection, and in some ways a magnification, of what you see in society, both good and bad. We are a nation of consumers, instant gratification and fast money. So, a logical step as a reflection of society is to use kids to make money and build reputations. The shoe and apparel companies are concerned with the bottom line. Sport stars sell shoes. With sports on 24/7 the kids imitate their role models, good and bad. We live in a throwaway world—be a national champion at 13, nobody at 16. Who cares? Essentially we, the adults, parents, coaches and administrators, have created a monster. What we see in today's kids is the result of an over-indulgent culture. We have lowered the bar, eliminated behavioral expectations and compromised sound educational principles to chase a pot of gold at the end of the rainbow that is not there for most.

So is it all that bleak, all gloom and doom? No way! We need to stop and take a long look at what we, as parents, coaches, administrators, and all adult authority figures need to do. We need to raise the bar, and set a higher level of expectation for the kids in areas that matter. I see the kids that I work with day-to-day achieve at a very high standard, just like the kids I coached 40 years ago. I have the same standards. The kids know what they are and consequently, reach up to those standards.

Let's stop blaming the kids and look at ourselves in the context of society. These kids are crying out for teaching, structure, and firm, fair discipline. They want the special experience that real coaching can provide. Let's not cop out and blame the kids. We all need to look in the mirror and raise our standards.

Train, Don't Strain

Training is just that, training—not an end unto itself.
Training is a mindful pursuit of specific goals intended to prepare

you for competition. Anybody can work hard. If every workout is a test of courage, or a time to put your back to the wall so that you end up being sick, then it is not training. Training is a cumulative process. There has to be a yin and yang to what you do. Hard days followed by easy days. Adaptation takes time. If you are straining through every workout, then there is a high probability that the adaptive response will be negative.

Remember, one workout cannot make an athlete, but one workout can break an athlete.

That Time of Year

This is a special, and in some ways, magical time of year for those of us who are involved in track and field as coaches or athletes. This is the championship season—the conference, state, regional and national championships. This is the time of year that all the training is pointed toward, the peak competitive season, the time when you reap the fruits of your labor. It is a time of great anticipation and doubt. Doubt, because you have more time to think: Have I done enough or have I done too much?

The really cool part is that it will all come out on the track or in the field. You have to lay it on the line. As a coach it is your final exam. I remember one of my athletes at Cal setting a personal best in javelin in our dual meet against Stanford, getting the measurement and running back down the runway and yelling, "I am peaking, I am peaking." She was and she did, going on three weeks later to win the AIAW national championship in the heptathlon.

This is the time of year when I really miss being a track coach. I have many great memories of the joy and the disappointment from meets like the Masters Meet in CIF Southern Section and the California State meet. For those of you who are coaching track now, enjoy it, be confident in your preparation and let the athletes perform.

Do You Talk Too Much?

Well, do you talk too much? This is a coaching disease.
Coaches love to talk and love to hear themselves talk. I know I love to talk. How else could I do 16-hour seminars by myself? Is what you are saying being heard? I just finished reading a book about Harvard crew called, *The Eight: A Season in the Tradition of Harvard Crew* by Susan Saint Sing (2010). You can't write about Harvard crew without writing about the legendary coach Harry Parker, an icon in the sport and a true coaching legend. Here is an observation by the author after one practice:

> There is largely silence. Harry has probably spoken fewer than a hundred words the entire practice. What he does mostly is watch. What the crews do mainly is wait for him to speak—and they execute.

John Wooden was the same way: one-phrase corrections with specific directions, no sermons, but short, sharp, exact and to the point. As a reformed screamer I have learned that tone of voice is also important. If you are yelling and screaming all the time, the athlete will quickly tune you out. Know what you have to say, say it, reinforce it and let the athletes execute. Empower them. After all, they have to do it not you. Remember, many times what you don't say is as important as what you do say. Ultimately, your effectiveness as a coach comes down to your ability to communicate. It is not what you say, it is what they hear. It is not what you show, it is what they see. Learn to say more by speaking less.

Fail Forward

I learned in an interview with Craig Venter (of human genome fame) that he and his group have just created the first fully functioning, reproducing cell controlled by synthetic DNA. The statement in the interview that really got my attention was that 99 percent of the experiments in the project had failed! 99 percent! I immediately thought that without the lessons learned from those failures, the project would never have succeeded.

There are many lessons here for us as coaches and teachers. Redefine failure as a learning opportunity. Push the envelope. As Tom Peters, the management consultant guru says, fail forward. Learn from your mistakes and failures and keep moving in the direction of the goal. Remember, to reach the goal it must be crystal clear—you need a fully functioning compass oriented to true north, along with an up-to-date map, to help you stay on course.

Speed

The sad part of speed is that so many people train it out of their athletes. I see this especially with the endurance athletes, but I even see it with speed and power athletes. It is about quality not quantity. Start with warm-ups. Some of these elaborate hour-and-fifteen-minute warm-ups that include every drill under the sun are just getting the athlete tired and not ready for explosive effort. Speed is about quality and economy of effort. I quote my good friend and colleague Gary Winckler, "Work capacity is not a biomotor quality." Speed is a quality that must be trained year round regardless of the event or sport discipline. The high neural and coordinative demands require that those pathways stay open and stimulated. Everyone has potential for speed, but many do not reach it because of improper training, or the belief that it cannot be improved.

Speaking of speed, I am reminded of James Thomas "Cool Papa" Bell. He was a star in the Negro Leagues and one of the fastest players to ever play the game of baseball. Sam Harriston, who was a coach with the White Sox when I worked there, had played with Papa Bell and he told this story to illustrate how fast he was. He said he was rooming with Papa Bell and they were both in their beds with the lights on in their room. Papa Bell got up to turn the lights off and was back in his bed before the lights went off. (I know this story is attributed to Muhammad Ali, but it was really Papa Bell). That is speed!

A Story and a Lesson

I have been thinking more about the lessons I have learned along the way in middle distance and distance training. I want to start out by saying that I have a clear bias toward the speed and the power influence. From speed and power will come more efficient mechanics and optimum force into the ground.

Middle distance and distance runners are not just big hearts and lungs with legs attached. There has be a convergence—a synergy, if you will—with all systems of the body working at the same time, together, to produce the desired speed for the intended distance.

Now to the story and the lesson. I think it was early February 1973, a Sunday morning around nine o'clock. I was warming up for a pole vault session at the UCSB (University of California, Santa Barbara) track. It was cold. The temperature was in the upper 30s (yes, it does get cold in California). I got there early to do some extra warm-up before meeting the coach who was helping me in the vault. Just I was going to begin my warm-up jog, Jim Ryan showed up. He asked me if he could jog with me. I thought to myself, you are asking me? I should be privileged just to be on the same track with you!

So we started our warm-up at my pace—a tendonitis trot, very slow at around an eight-minute mile pace. We did a mile. I was shocked. Jim sounded like a Hoover vacuum cleaner. His breathing was heavy, and his footfalls were loud and percussive. I knew he was having problems with asthma, but this seemed weird.

We stopped and did a few leg swings, a couple of stretches and then went to the infield to do "strides", 100-meter buildups opening up the stride. He was being polite and letting me set the tempo. The first two were slow—around 16 seconds for 100 meters. The same response happened just like when we were jogging—breathing heavy, with percussive foot strikes. Then I picked it up and dropped to around 14 seconds per hundred and then a couple around 13. Everything changed. It was a magical transformation. His breathing was quiet, his foot strikes were efficient, everything smoothed out. It was that beautiful, flowing, long, efficient stride that I'd seen so many times.

We stopped and chatted for a few minutes and he went off on a run. I have never forgotten that morning. I remember going home and puzzling over it. Why? Over the years I have seen this phenomenon repeat itself in so many ways. There was a point of physiological, neural and biomechanical convergence where all his systems were synced up and efficient. For him, it was a 15-second, 100-meter tempo, four-minute pace. At that speed everything came together in a finely tuned rhythm. So for me, the lesson I want to share with you as coaches, is to help the athlete find that rhythm, key in on it, and train it in. Don't plod and force unusually slow tempos on the athlete that are uncomfortable and inefficient. In my opinion and experience the same is true in swimming and cycling. Don't misinterpret this and take this out of context. I know you can't run fast all the time, but be aware of this convergence zone. Look for it and tap into it and you will get more out of what you do.

Middle Distance and Distance Training Thoughts

From the day I started coaching I have always approached the middle distance and distance events from a speed and power perspective. Very quickly I saw that those who could run forever, but could not run fast, were not going to be competitive in races. Remember, the winner is the person who can maintain the highest percentage of their maximum speed for the duration of the race. If you have speed and you want to be successful, then you must learn how to use your speed. The only way you learn to use it, is to run fast—train speed in, don't train speed out. Some fast running must be included during all phases of the training year.

Isn't this all about preparing the athletes to race? In my opinion there is too much emphasis on pace. Pace is a misleading term. It is not pace, it is distribution of effort. Distribution is what allows you to use the highest percentage of maximum speed for the duration of the race. Good distribution demands great and efficient running mechanics and the ability to change tempos (shift gears) in one stride. To learn race distribution you need to know your strengths and weaknesses and how you can run your race. You must become race hardened. That is a key element that is missing today. Without dual meets and smaller meets the young, developing runner is denied the opportunity to learn how to race and become race hardened.

Good running mechanics don't come from drills. Drills are part of the picture. Greater improvement in running mechanics comes from proper strength training. You must strengthen the legs and hips; this is neglected in most middle- and long-distance training programs. Strength is the basis for speed and good running mechanics.

Training or Coaching?

Are you training your athletes or coaching your athletes? There is a clear distinction. Unfortunately, today I see much more training than coaching. Here are some distinctions between coaching and training, as I see them:

TRAINING—Focused on the result. Just get it done.
COACHING—Focused on the process, how it is done, making sure it is repeatable.

TRAINING—Self-centered, all about the trainer, the athlete can't do it without the trainer.
COACHING—All about empowering and teaching the athlete. Creating self-sufficiency rather than dependence.

TRAINING—Trainer has all the answers.
COACHING—Always gathering data from the training, fine-tuning and learning.

TRAINING—Lots of screaming, yelling, and "motivating."
COACHING—Purposeful, meaningful feedback and cues, communicating and teaching.

TRAINING—Focused on equipment; needs machines and apparatus to train.
COACHING—Focused on the athlete and the sport they are preparing for, and coaches accordingly. Uses what is needed and necessary, not bells and whistles.

TRAINING—Scattered, all over the place.
COACHING—Focused on the task at hand. No cell phone!

TRAINING—Follows the latest fads, listens to gurus.
COACHING—Knows best practice and follows it. Stands on the shoulders of giants. Has a mentor.

I think this gives you the idea. Which are you? Look at yourself and look at your colleagues. If you are a trainer, become a coach. Coaching is much more satisfying and rewarding.

More Thoughts on Coaching and Training

Training contains a fair amount of redundancy. Use that to your advantage as a consistent means to compare and track progress. I know for years I have used a consistent pattern of warm-up that provides instant feedback for the athletes' training readiness for that day. The same goes for certain drills and workouts that I place simultaneously in a training cycle. As the athlete gains training age, this information becomes increasingly more valuable.

The best basis for future planning is careful contextual analysis of prior training. Therefore, it is very important to keep detailed training records and logs.

Don't always look for cause and effect; look for connections.

Use Foster's RPE rating. Wait for 30 minutes after the workout, then have the athlete rate the session on a 1-to-10 scale. Multiply that score by the minutes in the workout.

Talk less, listen more. Speak with meaning. The power in verbal communication often is not the words; it is the space between the words. The rhythm and pacing—how you say things—goes a long way to determine how and if the message is received.

As Martha Graham said, "Nobody cares if you can't dance well. Just get up and dance. Great dancers are not great because of their technique, they are great because of their passion." So let that passion flow through everything you do and say.

Role of Sport Science and Sports Medicine

Sport science is important in advancing our knowledge of training. I am a huge supporter of sport science, and during my career I have had the opportunity to work with some of the best practitioners. But sport science and the sport scientist do not captain the ship, the coach does. The same with sport medicine. Under that term I put the physio (ATC—Certified Athletic Trainer), physical therapist, chiropractor and doctor. They are important, but they should not captain the ship.

The captain of the ship should be the coach. The coach is the ultimate authority on what needs to be done to get his individual or team into the performance arena in optimum condition to perform. This means the coach must be a great communicator and organizer. The coach must be knowledgeable enough in sport science and sport medicine to be able to direct, detect, and ask the correct questions. I have seen first hand what happens when sport science or sport medicine runs amok and it is not pretty. The athlete suffers, the coach loses games and matches, the athletes underperform and no one is willing or able to take responsibility.

The performance team is the team behind the team. They should be invisible. There are no super-star sport scientists, or sport medicine practitioners. There are only star athletes and great teams. The spotlight should be on the athlete, not the support team. Let's just make sure that we have the horse before the cart, and the coach is driving the cart.

Creativity and Coaching

I view coaching as a very creative process. It would be interesting to see scientists study coaching as a creative process. In a trite manner we talk about the art and science of coaching, and then lean toward the science. I love the science of coaching, but I absolutely embrace the art. That is where the passion is, the fire in the belly, that joy of enhancing the dance of athletic movement. Too much science and we begin to view movement too mechanistically. We lock ourselves into artificial methods, modes and prescriptions unrelated to the big dance—the game, the match, the race. The creative coach will look at the same movement and see it with different eyes.

I will never forget presenting a movement analysis of the javelin in one of my graduate classes at Stanford. I presented the analysis in a very segmented, mechanistic manner, broken into parts, with a detailed analysis of each segment. I analyzed the film frame by frame, with no connection of one frame to the next. That is how I coached, frame by frame. When I finished, the graduate dance students in the class asked me to play the film loop again without stopping. I did. They asked me to play it again and then another time. On the fourth time I played it, they started clapping the rhythm. They saw the throw as a dance. What an aha moment! I honestly have to say a whole new world opened up for me that day. Movement is a dance, a jazz riff, and coaches are creative artists. It changed the way I looked at movement, and it changed the way I coached.

Opening the Door

In 1954, Roger Bannister broke the four-minute barrier in the mile. Bannister happens to be one of my sporting heroes. I think it is amazing that he did this while he was a full-time medical student. Because of his studies, he could only train for one hour a day. I read his book, The *Four-Minute Mile* when I first started coaching. That was when everyone was espousing super-high mileage, 150 miles a week plus. Bannister and his coach/advisor Franz Stampfl (read his book *Franz Stampfl on Running*—a coaching classic) had a program that nailed it. They trained for the race. I think there are many lessons we can learn from Bannister.

Lesson One: Have a life. If you just train, it is easy to take every little setback and blow it out of proportion.

Lesson Two: Train for your race—not only the race, but *your* race. Learn how you need to run or swim the distance based on your physical qualities.

Lesson Three: Stress quality. Any stumblebum can run miles or swim yardage. It is what you put into the miles that count—be efficient, do not waste steps.

Lesson Four: There are no barriers, just bigger targets to aim for. Four minutes proved to be a mental, not a physical barrier.

Lesson Five: Forget facilities and ideal training environments. Get out there and go for it. Train where you can. Create your own environment of excellence. The track where Bannister trained and set the record was far from an ideal training venue.

Lesson Six: Believe in yourself and know yourself. Have a coach/advisor and a support group you trust.

Lesson Seven: Don't listen to naysayers. Follow the path you choose and do not let anyone discourage you.

Turning Potential into Performance and Identifying Talent

Dan Coyle, author of *Talent Code*, writes:

> … *We fail at talent identification because we're looking in the wrong place. We instinctively look at performance (which is visual, measurable) instead of mindset and identity, which are what really matter, because they create the energy that fuels the engine of skill acquisition. They are the nuclear power-plant for the 10,000 hours of deep practice. They are the ghosts in the machine.*

The bottom line is: Look for that growth mindset—the little, scrawny kid who refuses to give up, who keeps coming back for more. Early in my coaching career a wise old coach told me that many are called and few are chosen.

In my years of coaching I have seen so many athletes with potential that has been unfulfilled. They were labeled early on as the next great ones. What happens? How can we get the athlete to realize their potential? In so many cases, potential, especially being identified as a prodigy early, can be a curse. But isn't it our jobs as coaches to help athletes understand and reach their potential? We can do this by focusing on the process rather than the outcome. We are better off praising effort rather than results, which is right out of Carol Dweck's book, *Mindset: The New Psychology of Success*.

I know I struggle with athletes who have been identified early as the next great one. I guess I identify more with the average athlete who has to fight and claw their way for everything they get. Potential seems to dull persistence. I saw this in the last couple of years with a team I was coaching. The player with the most potential did not achieve at the same level as her less talented teammates; in fact they began to pass her. I am not sure what the answer is here. I do know that it is a major part of my job as a coach to help translate potential into performance.

Fear Of Success

Everyone talks about fear of failure. I really do not think that is what it is. It is really fear of success. I am convinced that coaches and athletes fear success more than they fear failure. With success comes pressure. The more success you achieve, the more you are expected to succeed and the more pressure there is. Successful people do not fear failure. They use it to learn, and view it as a growth opportunity. They internalize it and use it to improve.

Unsuccessful people avoid succeeding like the plague. They know that by succeeding, expectations for success will rise. They are comfortable being mediocre. If you listen to their self-talk and chatter you will hear it. They usually have every excuse in the book why they can't be better. They also can tell you a million reasons why others who are succeeding are doing things they can't or won't do. These are the people that Carol Dweck has identified as those with a fixed mindset. Successful people have a growth mindset. They embrace challenges, and look at failure as a growth opportunity. They understand there will be missteps, but each of those is a learning opportunity. Embrace the pursuit of excellence; don't be afraid of it. To be the best is not comfortable. Everyday you have to go where few others dare to venture.

There is an American Dream

I just finished reading *American Victory—Wrestling, Dreams, and A Journey Toward Home* by Henry Cejudo with Bill Plaschke. I love stories like this. To me it proves there is an American dream. Henry's mother and father were illegal immigrants. His father abandoned the family when he was five-years old. His mother eventually got a green card through one of the amnesty programs. To say that this guy overcame every disadvantage possible to become an Olympic gold medalist does not begin to describe it. It is certainly an inspiring story. Have a dream and pursue that dream. Do not let anything stand in your way.

Some quotes from the book:

"To be the best, you've got to best the best, so why not start right now?" He said this when learning that he was to face the 2006 world champions in his first Olympic match.

What his coach at the USOTC (United States Olympic Training Center), Terry Brand, told him that inspired his post work-out routines that sometimes lasted an hour! "You've go to do something that nobody else in the world is doing, and you've go to do it everyday."

Practice pays off. The following was his comment on using the high crotch takedown, the move that won him the gold medal: "The perfect high crotch takedown. The approximately one millionth high crotch takedown. It is a move I had been doing hundreds of times a week for four years in practice. I could do it in my sleep. Now I just did it in my dream."

On the gold medal five ounces:
"A dozen years of sweat for five ounces."

Sport does not exist in isolation, it reflects society. Henry Cejudo did not use his background as an excuse. He gained strength and inspiration from it and channeled his misfortune into his training and performance. Success does not happen by chance!

The Training Session

The individual training session is the cornerstone of training. A long-term plan is a succession of linked individual training sessions in pursuit of specific objectives. It is the individual training session where the long-term plan is actually implemented. Therefore, it is important to understand the necessity of adjustments and flexibility within the context of the plan, especially at the level of the daily training session. Contingency planning is very important, and a necessary part of the planning process.

Every component in the workout must be in pursuit of the specific objectives of the workout and follow the general theme for that particular session. The workout is not an end in itself. It is a means to an end. Therefore it must be put in the context of the whole training plan, so it is important to not let the individual training session get blown out of proportion.

Coaching Excellence: Professional Development

How much time do you devote each day and each week to your professional development? I know one international federation in another country that spends 30 percent of their budget on professional development. I know I try to spend 45 minutes to an hour a day on professional development.

Joe Vigil, Ph.D, a great coach and mentor, does an hour of professional development reading, each morning at 5:00 A.M. He has been coaching for over 60 years and is now 80-years old. You are never too old or too knowledgeable to stop learning.

What exactly is professional development? First, I do not count time on the Internet reading trash. However, time on Internet sites related to coaching does count. They challenge you and make you think. Second, read books and research articles in and out of your field. Read authors that challenge your thinking. I try to read 100 books a year. Subscribe to periodicals and scientific journals. Third, interact with other professionals, attend conferences, and take trips to observe other professionals you respect. Fourth, invite other professionals to come and evaluate your work, as they will see things you miss.

Never stop learning and challenging yourself to improve. Just about the time you think you have it figured out, some new ideas will arise to challenge you. Stay ahead of the curve, and be proactive. Do not copy and follow, innovate and lead. The only way you can do this is through continual professional development.

> *Read, every day, something no one else is reading. Think, every day, something no one else is thinking. Do, every day, something no one else would be silly enough to do. It is bad for the mind to be always part of unanimity.*
> — Christopher Morley, American author and journalist

Mental Toughness

Mental toughness is a cop-out. I believe mental discipline trumps so called mental toughness all the time. All the champions I have been around had incredible mental discipline. Making someone sick in a workout or running someone until they drop does not build mental toughness. Find out who will do the workout when no one is there to make them do it. Find out who shows up and brings their "A" game every day no matter what the conditions and the circumstances. Those are the people who have mental discipline. Those are the people I want on my team.

Kettlebell Training

I do think some of the claims made for kettlebell training are a bit over the top. If you are training to do more reps with kettlebells or to express more strength with a kettlebell in a kettlebell competition, then by all means just train with a kettlebell. If not, look at the kettlebell method as one method among many that you can utilize. There are no Russian "secret" kettlebell training methods, as current marketing hype would lead you to believe.

Kettlebells were the staple of training in gyms and physical education in the late nineteenth and early twentieth centuries in the United States and in Europe. Just like medicine balls, climbing ropes, Indian clubs, and various other forms of apparatus training, they fell out of favor as physical education changed and moved away from movement gymnastics toward team sports. There has been revived interest in the last ten years as kettlebells have become commercially available for purchase. The ease of availability has been a major factor in their resurgence. It was a mode of training I have been familiar with since the beginning of my coaching career, but it was not a viable option because we could not get kettlebells. They were either unavailable or too expensive to ship from Europe.

The Pitch

No not a pitch, but the field in soccer. One day I was channel surfing and watched a few minutes of a game from the English Premier League. It was played on a beautiful pitch as flat as a billiard table, the grass closely manicured. The game was fast and exciting. The ball bounced true. Contrast that to an MLS (Major League Soccer) game on another channel. That game was played on an American football field. There was a crown on the field for drainage, and the field was full of divots. How can you play quality high-level soccer on fields not suited for the game? Yes, you need quality players, but there are more of those now in the U.S. Maybe we need to look at the obvious—how about the pitch?

Jim Radcliffe on Planning and Periodization

Jim Radcliffe, Head Strength & Conditioning Coach at the University of Oregon, has a great analogy for the process of planning.

> If we are going on a trip together, first we determine the destination. Then we decide how we want to get there and how many stops we want to make along the way for food and rest. It is different if it is a group. Then we have to have everyone on the bus and make sure the bus driver knows the destination and recognize that there will probably be more stops along the way to eat and go to the bathroom.

This is a simple but effective analogy. Let's not make the process of planning and periodization more complicated than that! Know your destination, recognize that there are different routes to get there and some will take longer than others.

Dinosaur or Cockroach: Adapted or Adaptable?

Do not look for adversity, look for opportunity. Ask yourself what you can do each day to make your athletes better. Carefully study the movements of the sports—understand the forces and how they are produced and reduced—and train accordingly. Get away from artificial limiting beliefs about what the body cannot do. Focus on the infinite possibilities that the body presents to solve movement problems. Train movements to enhance coordination and efficiency of movement. The body is completely adaptable. It has an amazing ability to compensate and solve movement problems. Yes, I said compensate. Great athletes are great compensators, and it is okay!

Artificial, sterile environments or strict, "correct" movements do not expand the body's ability to adapt to the demands of the sport. Sterile and artificial training environments and scenarios result in adapted bodies that cannot change and adjust to the random and chaotic demands of the sport. Open, challenging, movement-enriched environments create adaptable athletes who are able to adjust and modify movements on demand. These adaptable athletes, given a level of talent, are high performers and stay injury free.

Which would you prefer if you were to choose an athlete for competition? Do you want a dinosaur type who is completely adapted and on their way to extinction, or a cockroach type of athlete who is thriving and highly adaptable? I know who I want. I want the cockroach who can adapt to any environment under any circumstances. Ask yourself, are you training your athletes to be dinosaurs or cockroaches? I want adaptable athletes who can solve any movement problem presented to them.

Great Quote from a Great Athlete

Karch Kiraly, acknowledged to be the greatest male volleyball player ever, won two gold medals indoors and one outdoors on the beach. When asked how he prepared to win Olympic gold, he replied, "I never did. I only prepared to win the next play." This is a great message for coaches and for athletes.

Thoughts after Blogging 1,000 Posts

This blog is about sharing knowledge and provoking thoughts to define the field of athletic development. The following are some thoughts for you:

- Family and friends are first.

- We all stand on the shoulders of giants. We must honor and respect those who have gone before us and paved the way in order to make the journey easier for us.

- Often it is what you do *not* say, or do *not* do, that is as important as what you do say and do.

- Communication is a two-way process—sending and receiving. Lest we forget, it is not what we say or write, it is what we read or hear that ultimately determines the quality of communication.

- The body is not a machine. A reductionist, mechanistic approach will lead to segmented, robotic movement.

- Mistakes and losses are learning opportunities. Take advantage of them.

- In life we have three time zones—past, present and future. The past is gone. We should learn from it and move on, not dwell on it. We can take care of the future by doing a great job in the present.

- Knowledge and information are not the same.

- Coaching and training are not the same.

• Anyone can work, but does the work have purpose and direction?

• Simplify. Simplicity yields complexity.

Hopefully, there will be thousands more posts, as I challenge myself daily to gain knowledge and understanding. In turn, I will challenge you to do the same. For me this blog is just part of a longer journey on the functional path. It is certainly a journey worth traveling—a collection of experiences to be enjoyed and shared. Thanks for joining me on this journey.

Why? Why Not?

Why does the Newtonian, mechanistic, reductionist approach that focuses on minutiae and the parts persist? Why not a quantum approach that focuses on relationships and connections, flow and rhythm? I think the former is comfortable because it allows people clearer definitions. In some ways it is simplistic because really all you have to do in that approach is be a technician. If you understand how all the muscles work, what inhibits, what lengthens, what you need to activate and then what you need to integrate, it all fits into a neat, clean, little box. Just follow the algorithm and push a few buttons and everything is fixed.

Unfortunately, or fortunately, it is not that easy. The body is a self-organizing, chaotic system that is highly adaptable. It responds both negatively and positively to use and disuse. It is definitely not a machine. As coaches, trainers, therapists and doctors we must recognize the wisdom of the body, and train or treat accordingly. The best way to understand and assess movement is to get the body moving. Closely observe and feel how things connect and how they disconnect. Explore the dimensions that the wisdom of the body offers.

As coaches we must prepare the body for the demands of the sport. We do that by stressing the body to and beyond its limits at times. If we do that in a systematic and sensible manner, the body will adapt and thrive in the competitive environment. If we train not to be hurt and put limits on the body in training, then the body will not be ready for the extreme demands of the actual competition. We are doing a disservice to athletes with a benign approach.

No Instructions Included, Just Play

Recognize and use the wisdom of the body. The body is very smart; instinctively it knows what to do. It gets confused when we put artificial restraints on it and it rebels by getting hurt or not performing to optimum levels. No instructions needed or included; just some common sense and a feel for movement, and then go play.

Let the Coaches Coach

Today, what we have going on in professional sport, and to a certain extent in collegiate sport, is alarming to me. The prevalence of the so-called medical model with the team doctor sitting at the top of the pyramid, the physical therapist next, followed by the team trainer, and then last in the pecking order, the strength and conditioning coach. There are many situations when every exercise—I truly mean every exercise—must be approved by the team medical staff before the strength and conditioning coach can implement a program.

Frankly, this is pretty ridiculous; it is actually a formula for failure. Sure, there must be accountability, but accountability works both ways. I vividly recall my meeting with a team doctor like it was yesterday. He was questioning some exercises we were doing, and had been doing with no problems for nine years. My admonition to him was, "I do not tell you how to do surgery, so do not tell me how to do exercises." Doctors are not trained in exercise; it is not part of their skill set. There needs to be mutual respect, professionalism and accountability for all concerned.

I really think the blame for this must be shared. There are strength and conditioning coaches who are in the dark ages. They are one dimensional; they never leave the weight room. Many of the coaches in pro sports are afraid of players and are unwilling to push them or demand accountability from them. The approach is to do as little as possible, and to avoid hurting them or making them tired in case they complain to the trainer, or worse, to management or their agent.

I am amazed at the level of naiveté with which the teams approach conditioning and injury prevention. Now we have situations where all the players do is roll on foam rollers, and do ridiculous sequences of exercises that have fancy objectives like inhibit, lengthen, activate, and integrate. They do this as "training" and wonder why they have injuries. How about designing a good training program that gets them moving and gets them functionally fit, fast and strong for their sport?

Scott Boras, the baseball agent—probably the most powerful agent in sport—gets it. In an article titled, "Who's in Charge Here?" published in the Oct. 8, 2007 issue of *ESPN The Magazine*, Matthew Cole writes:

> *As a former player, Boras believed that owners didn't invest enough in their talent, their product. Teams treated players like replaceable parts. They had pitchers and shortstops do the same training, the same lifting and stretching. It didn't make sense. The teams didn't start teaching players how to stay healthy and fit until they were men, which shaved years off performance. Not for this kid, Boras told himself.*
>
> *"Imagine adding seven years to your career," Boras tells his new kids. Imagine what history you can make with those years. Boras shows them the batting cages and the private gym. This is an*

institute, not some spa. Each member of Team Boras gets a dedicated program designed by Steve Odgers, the former White Sox conditioning director and decathlete, who has a neck the width of an oak tree, a guy with 13 years of training data etched in journals. Odgers gets prospects when they're just out of high school and puts them through a year-round program designed specifically for each player—because a relief pitcher is not the same as a second baseman. He even teaches them yoga. Show me a team that can do all that. Throughout the year, Boras dispatches Odgers and four other trainers around the country to check in on A-Rod, Dice-K, Pudge and the rest. It's Odgers who tells teams what program the players should follow. Boras knew he couldn't call trainers himself—they'd never listen to a moneyman, but one of their own, that's a different story. And if a team's trainer squawks about outside interference, Boras might pick up the phone and call the GM.

He knows what he has to do to prolong the careers of his players. Why can't the teams figure it out? The medical model is not the answer.

Program Design

I always start out with the finished product in the forefront of my mind. It must be clear what we want to achieve at the end of the training program. I want to make sure that deficits are addressed. I want to make sure that threads of all components of training are always there, that nothing disappears or gets lost in the shuffle. I try to have a theme for each cycle and specific objectives for each session. I want the objectives to be measurable.

I always try to incorporate variability without creating confusion. For example, with volleyball, the variability will come from derivatives of exercise and drills rather than introducing an entirely new drill. I am always aware of context. I want to make sure the athlete is being sufficiently challenged so that there will be training adaptation. Rest and recovery are important both intra-workout and inter-workout. Unfortunately, at the high school level, intersession recovery is out of my control. I confer closely with the coach to understand the content of the technical and tactical work. I attend each session so that I can make any adjustments necessary based on what I see during practice.

In regard to planning the actual session, that is the key to the whole process. The warm-up tends to become pretty mundane, so I work to cycle that according to the time of the season. It is very important because it is what transitions them from their daily activities to training and it sets the tempo for the session. Also, it gives me feedback as to soreness or possible modifications I must make in the session. In setting up sessions I have a rule I call the 3 x 6 rule—three training tasks in six minutes—high intensity, quality reps. For the last activity of the session I follow the "Winckler Law." My colleague Gary Winckler, formerly women's track coach at the University of Illinois, gave me this idea years ago: Make the last thing you do in a session have a training effect that is similar to the way you want them to start the next session. Therefore, I always end with some quick, fast and explosive work so that is what they remember for the next session. Simple, but effective. I hope these ideas stimulate you to think about how you design your training.

It Comes Down to SPEED

Haile Gebrselassie broke the marathon world record in Berlin in 2008, with an official time of two hours, four minutes and twenty-six seconds. At the half way mark he was at 1:02:29. He had his fastest kilometer split of 2:50 at 35 K. It all comes down to speed. The winner will always be the person who can sustain the highest percentage of their maximum speed for the race distance. Look at this guy's track times. Anyone who thinks distance running is about pounding long, slow miles needs to rethink their approach. I have always loved to watch this guy run because I felt he was the model of running efficiency, with a very compact stride that enabled him to instantly change gears.

Old School

What exactly is old school? Is it old school to have a work ethic? Is it old school to respect your opponents and your teammates? Is it old school to respect your coach? Is it old school to make a tackle and get up and go back to the huddle—no celebrations or sack dances? Is it old school to have to pay your dues? It is old school to take responsibility for your actions? Is it old school to just play the sport because you love competing—no worry about earning a scholarship or being ranked on Web sites as one of the top players in the country?

Let's all wake up! We are all party to this—the athletes, coaches, parents, administrators, and the media. Let's get back to basics and enjoy sport for the essence of it. Let's put play and fun back into sport. We can't turn back the clock, but we can take a look in the mirror and see what each of us can do to change what is happening.

Basic Paradigm for Program Evaluation

This is a paradigm I have used for years. It has worked well for me and my colleagues. I truly believe that by applying this paradigm and understanding the basic principles of training, that you should be able to work effectively with any sport. Here it is:

1. Know the demands of the game or sport.
2. Know the demands of the position or event.
3. Know the qualities of the individual athlete.
4. Know the pattern of injuries in the sport.

Over the years I have found that if I deviate from this, there will be problems. Once I have gone through the evaluation of these four steps, then it is a matter of determining the need-to-do versus the nice-to-do training activities. This simple paradigm will allow you to derive as complex a training program as is needed.

This paradigm really evolved when I was working as Al Vermeil's assistant at the Chicago Bulls in the mid-'80s. I thought that some of the things I was having the players do in regard to conditioning were not really based on the game of professional basketball, so I went to Al to get the video guy to shoot individual, isolated video of our top six players in games. What a revelation! It was not basketball; it was more like football or wrestling. It certainly made me rethink my ideas about conditioning for pro basketball.

I do not know what was done in regard to the Bulls, because I left soon after that to go to work for the White Sox. I know that with the White Sox we carefully studied the demands of the game, individual positions, and the individual players. It is all part of a comprehensive system of athletic development. With the sophisticated tools available today there is no excuse for what we see in regard to conditioning for various sports. The conditioning must fit the game, the position and the athlete, and must prevent injury. Too often we are trying to force the athletes into boxes. Things like the Big Three or distance running for speed power simply do not reflect the reality of sport demands. As the old cowboy used to say, you can lead a horse to water, but you can't make it drink.

You do not have to play the sport to know the sport. Today, there are many tools to use in order to learn a sport. Virtually every sport has instructional books and videos available that explain the sport from a technical and tactical perspective. Also, remember the rules of the sport also dictate conditioning. That is why high school, collegiate, and NFL football have subtle differences. To continue the American football example, something like a no-huddle offense will impact how you condition your offensive players. As far as having played the sport, especially at a high level, I do not feel it is important at all; in fact, it can be a hindrance. Not playing the game allows a completely unbiased perspective. I have found that many people who were stars think they did things one way when in actual practice they did it differently.

When looking at game demands I would use GPS and accelerometer data if available. This data enables the conditioning and strength training to be more exact and also specific to the individual athlete. Many people have used heart rate data extensively; personally, I have not put as much stock in this. I feel it is pretty predictable and there are too many artifacts in the data to base training solely on heart rate.

I think it is also important that the game itself and practice for the game, play a huge roll in actually conditioning the player. The game represents the highest form of stress. I know the good soccer coaches I have worked with have made practices very game-like so my emphasis was on speed, quickness and power development. Actual fitness was not as much of a consideration because of the types of practices they ran. John Wooden and Dean Smith are good examples of this in basketball.

As you work through all the steps of the paradigm you will see a true system begin to evolve. It is a both a scientific and an experiential process.

Stretching and Warm-up

It never ceases to amaze me how warm-up and stretching are equated. Warm up to stretch; do not stretch to warm up. There is plenty of research to show that pre-exercise stretching does not prevent injury. Despite this knowledge you still see football teams lying on the ground for ten minutes doing static stretching. What a waste. Don't get me wrong, there is a place for active stretching in warm-up, such as in the latter third of the warm-up when the body is well on its way to being warmed up. Watch Oregon football warm up. That is the way it should be done—active and dynamic. I have been using an active warm-up with a minimum of static stretching for thirty-plus years. I think the results and lack of injuries bear out its efficacy.

That is not to say that flexibility is not important; it certainly is. It is a question of *when* you work on flexibility. It is a separate and distinct training unit. It is best done postpractice or after a good warm-up.

Protecting the Pitcher?

Why protect, when we should be thinking build and develop? The athletes are only fragile because we make them fragile. You protect by being proactive—by doing the correct work to prepare to pitch. I strongly believe that we need to take a long, hard look at what has become the contemporary approach toward the development and training of pitchers. They are athletes, and should be coached and trained accordingly. Build them from the ground up. Stop emphasizing the arm and shoulder; they are the last links in the kinetic chain. Work on the whole kinetic chain.

The biomechanics of pitching have been thoroughly studied. Look closely at those studies. Don't listen to opinion. Look at scientific fact and develop the program accordingly. That is what we did with the White Sox almost 20 years ago. So far nothing has been discovered to refute what we did.

Work on mechanics without making pitchers so mechanical that they look like clones. At the developmental stages, teach them one pitch—the fastball. Learn how to command the strike zone with a fastball, and then learn a change-up instead of a breaking pitch. Breaking pitches should not be taught or allowed until at least the junior year of high school.

Institute a structured throwing program that includes throws at various distances and at varied intensities. Include one bounce throwing to a target to encourage rotation and correct and complete follow-through.

Building and training the pitcher is another means of protection. Artificial pitch count limits do not solve the problem—they actually contribute to it. The pitcher never learns how to adjust and pitch in a tough situation, and with a certain amount of fatigue. A good athletic development program will prepare them for the demands of pitching. Remember, to be better at anything you must practice that activity. To become a better pitcher, you must pitch.

Train Speed In or Train Speed Out

Speed is the most precious of all the biomotor qualities. It is dependent on fine motor control, coordination and explosiveness. That being said, training speed out of someone is simply emphasizing the type of training that negates those qualities. Speed and endurance are at opposite ends of the spectrum. You can train both, but not to the fullest extent of each at the same time. There must always be a thread of speed development work throughout a program in any sport. If you get too far away from speed then it is hard to get it back because it is such a neural quality. The concept of *training speed through endurance* is contradictory and basically fallacious. I conceptualize speed as an electric shock that excites the nervous system. For the middle distance and distance athlete—and any sport that has an endurance component—this is a good way to think about it. Use it wisely, do not overdo it, and remember that optimum speed development must have a foundation of good movement mechanics.

Let's not overcomplicate this. You coach speed into the athlete by training speed at the appropriate time in the workout, using an appropriate method and dosage for the time of the training year.

You train speed out by doing all sorts of general non-specific work and slow *base building* type of work. Remember you are what you train to be! To be fast you must train fast. When I hear a coach say that he or she has not started speed work yet, I just smile and hope we can compete against those teams often.

Thoughts on Speed Training from Stephan Widmer

Stephan is an outstanding sprint coach. He is the Head Coach of the Queensland State Swimming Centre in Brisbane, Australia. He coaches sprint swimmers, but the more I get to know him, the more I am convinced he could coach speed in any discipline. Here are some ideas that he presented on speed development at the ASCA (American Swimming Coaches Association) Convention in San Diego a few years back. It is interesting to note that he is a graduate of the Federal Technical Institute in Zurich, Switzerland. He has an excellent foundation in sport science, and also has the practical experience of being a top-class swimmer and a graduate of a program that required proficiency in at least ten sports (very much like our traditional physical education majors used to be in the States). I think regardless of the sport, you will find these common-sense ideas useful:

- Must have a passion for speed and power.
- Speed improves through skill.
- Attention to detail is necessary.
- Stresses to his swimmer, "How good is your worst repetition?"
- 3R's—Rhythm, Range and Relaxation.
- High level of concentration necessary and less space for error.
- Constant flow of energy and body parts.
- Specific training and race modeling necessary for sprint events (I could not help but think of Gary Winckler's race models here).
- Learn from TES (Top End Speed).

• Training needs to be distance specific in terms of Top End Speed (TES), Front End Speed (FES) and Back End Speed (BES).
• What is Back End Speed (BES) training without Front End (FES) stimulation?
• Must account for difference between genders.
• Start with speed. Early in the season the swimmers are fresh, so this is a perfect time for speed. Good time to feel speed and teach speed.
• Beware of training speed into the athlete versus training speed out of the athlete.
• Speed demands a high skill level and fast execution of precise movements.
• Train different speed zones.
• Energy system readiness rather than energy system emphasis.

In Spite Of, Not Because Of

Remember, above all else, talent will prevail. The cornerstone of a great program is a system of talent identification and acquisition. In the American non-system it is recruiting. Now you've got them, what do you do? Some people are smart enough to leave the athlete alone and let the talent rise to the top. This is very Darwinian and is typical in sports like professional baseball. The scary part is that sometimes the athletes are so talented that no matter what you do, they will prevail.

I went to a presentation at ASCA from the coach of an American record-holding sprint swimmer that blew me away. The weight-training program was right out of the 1970's—a body building program that Arnold would have been proud of. The swim program in the water training was more like what you would do with an open water swimmer. Truly amazing, but I see this all the time. Sure there are many roads to Rome—some are more direct and some more circuitous.

However, with our increasing scientific studies, we do know better. There are scientific principles that are not refutable, and there is also good practice. Neither can be ignored. I am amazed that people lose games because their players get slower and hurt, but there is never a connection made to training. It is particularly ironic that many of these people preach that they do not want to do anything in training that might cause the athletes to get hurt. They never sensitize them in practice to the demands of the sport, yet expect something miraculous to happen on Saturday or Sunday. Let's get real and pragmatic and take an educated, proactive approach to training the athletes we work with. Everyone can get better if aided by a systematic, sequential, and progressive training program.

Experience—More Thoughts

I am continually amazed at how experience is both undervalued and overvalued. It is overvalued because we get caught in the trap of thinking that experience is all about how many years rather than what went into the years. The coaches and professionals who I admire and emulate are the people who have had different experiences. They have tried new things and failed. They have pushed the boundaries and gotten out of their comfort zone. They have used their experience as a launching pad, not an anchor.

I spent a fair bit of time at the ASCA Convention with Nort Thornton, the men's swim coach at Cal Berkeley, who continues to coach there in his retirement. He is a prime example of a coach whose experiences are valued. He was attending presentations and taking notes. He is 75-years old and still learning and trying to improve what he does with swimmers. He has been an inspiration to me over the years because of his approach. Has he made mistakes? Sure he has, but he has learned from his mistakes and not repeated them over and over. He said something to me after a young coach had come up and commented to me that he wished I had shown more videos of exercises during my talk. Nort said, "They want the x's and o's but they don't know the why's. They all want the recipe but they have not yet learned how to cook."

I will close with a quote from *Texts and Pretexts* (1932) by Aldus Huxley, English critic and novelist, "Experience is not what happens to a man; it is what a man does with what happens to him."

Blocking Change and Innovation

Perhaps the two biggest and most frequently occurring blocks to change and innovation are two simple statements: "We already do that," and "Let me play devil's advocate." I have heard those two statements way too much. They lead to maintenance of the status quo and eventual stagnation. Obviously, if you already do something then there is no need to seek out change and innovation, but what if the things you are doing are not producing results? By playing devil's advocate, you are already thinking about why an idea cannot work instead of thinking about how it could work. Those are just a couple of thoughts for those of you who are working in an environment that stifles change and innovation. Sometimes being a change agent is not comfortable.

Following a Training Roadmap

Each journey is unique, even if the destination is not. Sometimes the weather will be clear, other times stormy. Sometimes construction or a special event may slow you down or steer you toward another route. If you're taking a fully loaded truck, you'll probably want to take a different route than if you have a sports car.

Similarly, no two athletes are the same. Even when it appears they're going to the same destination, they may need to get there via different routes. Each sport has unique demands, as does each position or event within a sport. Developing athletic performance is a complex process with seemingly endless variables in play.

However, to make the journey more manageable, you must look for similarities in movements and common characteristics between sports and individual positions. If you don't, the complexity will be too great. You'll either get lost entirely or revert to a one-dimensional training philosophy and trade effectiveness for simplicity.

Regardless of the destination, the most effective roads on the functional path are progressive and sequential, giving the athlete increasingly difficult movement problems to solve—a process known as adaptation. The body is highly adaptable, and if left to its own devices, will find a way to get the job done. We do not need a detailed script or a paint-by-numbers approach. That only stifles an athlete's creativity and limits their natural movement patterns. Still, you must have a well-planned progression that builds on previous gains to keep the athlete moving forward.

There will be speed limits, red lights, and construction zones along the way, all of which must be accounted for. While it may be tempting to ignore those limits, doing so may actually slow you down. You could end up being pulled over for speeding, find yourself breaking down, or get into an accident. Similarly, if you rush the adaptation process by having athletes try to lift too much too soon, or move on to more complex movements before mastering basic ones, you risk doing more harm than good. Only the proper progression will lead you to your ultimate athletic destination.

The "F" Word: Function

A colleague, Joe Przytula, wrote the following to me:

You used to use the phrase, "All training is functional training."
As a matter of fact, you once spoke of moving away from the
"F" word. Elaborate on what changed your mind, and if you still
stand by that quote.

Joe, I still stand by the quote, now more than ever. But as you know, it must be considered in context. What activity or exercise are you using relative to the desired outcome? I think of function as a continuum from 0 to 10—0 is death and 10 is the actual activity you are training for. If the majority of your training is not in the 7-to-10 range on the 10-point scale then you are lower on the continuum of function and it will probably take longer to achieve your goals, if in fact you do.

Yes, I tried to get away from using the words function or functional. Around late 2002/early 2003 I felt it all had become trivialized. Everything began to be called *functional training* or *functional rehab*. Of course, by my definition as stated above, that was correct, but it all became very confusing. It seemed that the weirder and more far out you could make the activity, the more *functional* it was. In many respects, this continues today. It has not reached its nadir. As a person who has been espousing this approach far longer than I would care to remember, I felt a debt of responsibility—and still do—to clarify and define, not to confuse and trivialize.

Some of my hesitancy to use the "F" word was an overreaction to an uncomfortable position I was put in at a clinic. I was explaining concepts and showing exercises and movements that represented what I espoused to be functional training. Everything that I showed had simple progressions that demanded mastery of one step before moving to the next step. That is the way I was taught, and I continue to teach this way. It was more than a hodge-podge of exercises and equipment.

For me, the straw that broke the camel's back was the fact that I was to follow a talk where the people lay on the ground and put a little mini cone on their bellies and tried to suck the cone in to learn the infamous *drawing-in maneuver*, the secret to core function. Then they would come to me and we would work through a progression of reaches and bends designed to feed through the core and lead to higher-level movements. This was all done standing and moving involving gait. The juxtaposition could not have been greater.

I chose to disappear for a while to get my bearings and make sure that I had not lost my compass. I stepped back and looked long and hard at my philosophy and the science behind what I believed in. I came to the conclusion that I had been on the right path, the *functional path*. I decided to retake the high ground and reclaim the use of the word in the context of what I believe it to be, regarding athletic development and rehab. That is my mission going forward— no hidden agendas, no impending certifications, just education and research to keep learning and moving ahead.

The Recipe

You can have all the ingredients of a great meal but without a cook who has a feel and touch for what they are doing, a clear vision of the finished meal, and good recipes to blend all the ingredients in a systematic manner, you have nothing. For good lessons in coaching watch the food channel!

WOW!

This comment was sent in regard to a post on hamstring injuries:

> Vern, running curves and arches could compromise the ankles of a player already playing his/her sport. Sprint straight ahead while training and leave the lateral movements to the sport itself.

This is exactly what has caused the problem. You must prepare for the demands of the game. Strength is only one piece of the puzzle. You must prepare for the torque involved and learn proper running technique, as it must be adapted to the game.

One of the reasons there are so many more injuries today than ever before is because they are taking that approach. You must train to play, not play to train! If these guys would take fifteen minutes a day and pay attention to preparation to play you would see a significant reduction in injuries. Instead, they all do a group stretch, jog a bit and declare themselves ready to rev up the engines. How many times have I heard, "I will turn it on when the lights come on?" A loser's lament.

The Madness of the Method

Air, water, dumbbells, smartbells, free weights, machines, altitude, submersion—use whatever you choose. All is for naught if it is not based on sound training principles grounded in sport science and proven practice. It is not the training methods or the exercise; it is the system. When and where does the method fit? When is it appropriate to include things? When is it inappropriate? How can the training effect be measured? The fact is that sound training requires direction and purpose. The goal of a systematic training program is to achieve results that can be consistently repeated.

Change

I have had several people ask me why baseball does not change. The comments were something like this: "After all, those are multi-million dollar players. Don't they want them to get better?" The answer is simple and it transcends baseball. In order to change you must want to change. Then you must make a sincere and total commitment to change. You have to wipe the slate clean and start anew. There are so many examples in the sport world, it is mind-boggling. American throwers fall flat on their faces in world championships. Why? Because their preparation and training are stuck in the past. It is about as contemporary as a Jefferson Airplane vinyl album. Alan Webb failed to medal—it was very predictable. He is trained to run for time, not to race. Change is constant and uncomfortable. To hang with the big dogs and perform at the highest levels, a high level of discomfort is demanded. Many are not willing to pay that price and many others do not know how to get there.

Nadal and Federer: Striving Together

The Latin derivative of the word competition is *competere*, to seek together. Roger Federer and Rafael Nadal epitomize this. To be a great champion you must have a worthy opponent to push you to greater heights. This is what these two men are doing. Here is an excerpt from an article in this week's (Aug. 27, 2007) *Sports Illustrated* titled, "Courtly Rivals," by L. Jon Wertheim that is very revealing about these two men:

> … And here's where their rivalry is different from most: There's not a trace of animosity in it. Each man is relentlessly differential toward the other, dispensing more props than a Broadway stagehand. Says Nadal, "To me he is the best player." Says Federer, "Trust me, I know how good Rafa is."
> Hearing them gush like this it becomes apparent they are not opposite after all. They were both raised in traditional European families that regard ego as a major character defect. Federer's modesty is as characteristic as his silken backhand. (He spent part of his last Christmas break visiting an orphanage in India.) But Nadal's not a prima donna either. At the French Open the two-time defending champ was spotted sweeping the clay courts when he was done practicing. "We're no better than anyone else," says his uncle and coach, Toni Nadal.

There are many lessons here for our spoiled American superstars. You do not have to trash talk and beat down your opponent to be the best. Let your performance do the talking. Seek out and relish worthy competition, and honor them. That is the essence of true sportsmanship.

Some Thoughts on Training

Real training is characterized by:

- No fads.
- No frills.
- Just training appropriate for the sport.
- Basic.
- Fundamental.

I have always said that it is essential to differentiate between the need-to-do and the nice-to-do. Yesterday, my colleague, Bill Knowles, gave me another to consider: The want-to-do.

A thought from John Wooden: "Things turn out best for those who make the best of the way things turn out."

Work or Training

I was talking to a swim coach the other day and he made the following comment: "I saw something on a Web site on kettlebell training and it looks really hard. I think I will put it in my program." I took a deep breath and admonished him to take a step back and think about what he was trying to achieve.

It is hard, but is it beneficial training in the context in which he wants to use it? Kettlebells until you are sick may make you tired but will it make you better?

Kettlebell work is a viable training method. It is not new and it was not invented to train the Russian Special Forces. In fact there was kettlebell training before there were Russian Special Forces. I do not see it as a focal point or a cornerstone of a training program. It is one piece of the training puzzle. In my estimation, there are many things that must be done to prepare and lead up to kettlebell work.

In my system it is a mode to achieve the following: Total body work—pulling movements; Upper body—pushing movements; and Core—swinging and chopping. As a mode of training it must fit the system, not the other way around. If you do not approach it that way, then the tail is wagging the dog.

There are secondary adaptations (I want to credit Carl Valle for this term) that occur with kettlebell training aside from the strength gains:

1. Increased proprioceptive demand.
2. Greater recruitment of synergistic and stabilizing muscles.
3. Greater metabolic coast? (Jury is out on this one.)

Use the mode in a system as part of a spectrum strength-training approach. One caution is that you can develop some wrist and elbow tendonitis if you do not use proper grip and technique.

Mr. Platehead

If you only look at the world through the hole in an Olympic weight plate, you will lose peripheral vision.
Continually looking at movement from one point of view becomes a self-fulfilling prophecy. Look at the big picture. Look at relationships and connections. How can these be enhanced and fostered? If there is

a problem, where is the breakdown occurring? Approach each training problem with a beginner's mind—have no preconceived notions. Think and look globally. See movement with different eyes. Be willing to take a risk. Try a new path. There is a big difference between a routine and a rut. Are you in a rut with your training programs? Remember, a tool in one person's hands can be a weapon in another's.

Losers' Laments

- I peaked too soon.
- I peaked too late.
- I never peaked.
- My periodization was too linear.
- My periodization did not undulate, but I did!
- I have not started speed work.
- Too much speed work.

How True

Is this not true in any sport?

Take a strong wrestler, get them tired, and they aren't as strong.
Take a quick wrestler, get them tired, and they aren't as quick.
Take a technical wrestler, get them tired, and they aren't as technical.
No matter what kind of wrestler, everyone is afraid of getting tired.
It's those who learn to perform when they're tired that find success.

- J. Robinson

Anyone can perform when they are fresh and rested, but the moment of truth in a game or match comes when the athlete can execute when they are fatigued. This is what we need to prepare our athletes for. Constantly prepare and condition for the moment when the game or match is on the line. That requires training that is mindful and meaningful—training with a purpose.

Entitlement or Paying Your Dues

This might be more appropriate for two old, broken-down coaches sitting on the front porch of a rest home talking about the good old days, but here goes: Just being there and putting in the time are not enough. Good enough is not good enough if you want to be the best. To be the best at what you do requires more than saying you are the best. You must pay your dues. Earn respect. Continue to learn. Never be satisfied.

I must admit, I am baffled by a lot of what I see today in the younger generations, especially generations Y and X. For some reason these generations seem to have a sense of entitlement. I have heard too many 30-something coaches complaining about the long hours and low pay, the time they must spend in the off-season—in short, all things that are part of earning your way. Wake up guys and gals. Pay your dues. Show your worth. Do not let other people define your jobs. You define them. Do the job better than anyone else. Prove your worth and then, and only then, will you get rewarded both professionally and financially. I asked someone the other day why he deserved a pay raise when the team is terrible and underachieving and there are too many injuries. I asked him what he had done to make the team better. The response was, "It is not my fault." Then whose is it? It is simple. If it is up to me, my fate is in my hands where it should be. Get up, get out, and get going. Seize the opportunity and prove your worth, and then the rewards will come.

Steve Nash

Steve Nash, a Canadian professional basketball player who plays point guard for the Phoenix Suns, is not a one-trick pony. During the summer he plays soccer. He plays on different recreation league teams in New York.

Nash spends most of the year running the point for the Phoenix Suns, but in the off-season, he can be found playing soccer in rec leagues in New York. "It's better for me than just running lines," he said. "I don't want to play a lot of basketball until September's over or I'll burn myself out. I just shoot, work out and play soccer."
("It's a Vision Thing for Nash in Soccer and in Basketball,"
NY Times, August 10, 2007)

I think there is a real message here that reinforces what many of us have been preaching—it is about having a base of athleticism and movement skills. He grew up in Victoria, Canada, playing a wide array of sports. He probably played more soccer than basketball in his youth. His brother is a national team player for Canada.

When I first saw Steve Nash, he was a high school junior at a private school in Victoria. I was the conditioning coach for the Canadian National Basketball Team at the time. Ken Shields, the head coach, invited him over to an evening practice and scrimmage with the National Team at Mount Douglas High School. He was not as tall and physically mature as he is now, but clearly you could see the potential and the athleticism. From then on, he polished and honed his basketball skills, but never forgot the athletic base. In testing during my time with the Canadian team, through 1994, he was by far the fittest player as measured on the Leger Beep test. Today, it is cool to want to be like Steve, but I am not sure everyone understands what he has done to get to where he is today.

One-Trick Pony

Are you training a one-trick pony? What do I mean? Essentially, are you putting all your eggs in one basket and emphasizing one component of a training method with your athletes? If you are, I would urge you to reconsider because that one trick will wear thin. Then what?

Rocky Had it Right

Was Rocky Balboa onto something when he was training in the meat locker? Current thinking would seem to indicate that he was ahead of his time. My friend Dean Benton, performance director for the Brisbane Broncos, said that if he had his way he would have the team spend halftime in a refrigerator truck. When he first mentioned this I thought he had lost it. Since then, I have come across this idea more and more. I've heard of a rugby team in England using a cold storage facility for recovery. I have read a couple of articles that suggest there is validity to this. Anecdotally, the comments that I hear are that the players feel refreshed. I have no idea of protocols or ideal temperature, but it certainly is thought-provoking. Will teams that are traveling ask the hotel to use their walk-in refrigerator? If I were a betting man I would say, yes.

Dancing on the Edge

Can a genius be satisfied with the mundane and the status quo? I was watching a documentary on movie producer and director Sam Peckinpah. His approach made me think about this. He was always dancing on the edge, pushing the envelope on what could be done in film. It got me thinking that this was also true in human athletic performance. To be the absolute best, you have to push the envelope; you must dance on the edge. The difference between high-level athletic performance and sickness and injury are akin to balancing on a razor's edge. It is almost like you have to be a gunfighter. You must be on the edge, living with the constant realization that there is always someone out there who could be faster.

I am convinced that is why so many athletes will not retire, and when they do, they have a tough transition to normal life. High-level competition and training is an almost constant rush, an adrenaline high necessary to get to the top and stay there.

Isolate or Integrate

I received the following query:

> *When do you isolate a joint or, in other words, when would the ankle complex need to get special exercises to ensure it's working properly, or when would the adductor/hammy complex need manual therapy to break up adhesions? Just curious as to what you do in actual practice.*

I try to avoid isolation at all costs. In my world, there is no place for isolation or reductionism. If the ankle joint needs special exercises we will work hard to devise movements that cause the ankle joint to dominate the movement, so we don't have to take another step to integrate it back into the system. If manual therapy is needed or based on a qualified medical opinion then I will not do anything. I will find the best qualified physical therapist that knows ART (Active Release Techniques) and ASTYM (a form of augmented soft tissue mobilization) and have them work on it. I am a coach, not a therapist. I work with great therapists as part of a performance team. Also, you seem to imply that movement is initiated by the core. Movement occurs around and through the core. It is not initiated by the core. Gait is the cornerstone of function. In short, what I do in practice is coach—no hidden agenda.

Words and Exercises

Words are just that, words. Words by themselves have meaning, but they do not have the same power until they are put in context. The same holds true for an exercise. An exercise is just that, an exercise, until it is put in context. This is a consistent theme that I continually try to emphasize.

Words and exercises represent a reductionist, isolationist approach.

Context represents the opposite—a big picture, integrated, quantum approach. It is so trite to say that the whole is greater than the sum of its parts, but it is so true. The process of building and rebuilding an athlete is not linear and reductionist. Rather, it is a process of never losing sight of the big picture, stressing coordination and integration.

Listen To Your Body

Coaches always tell the athletes to listen to their bodies. Do we ever tell them what they should listen for or listen to? What if they don't hear anything?

Entertainment, Not Sport

Does everything you see in professional sports today really surprise you? If it does, then you are pretty naïve. Professional sport is not sport; it is entertainment. I am not sure yet if it is a reality show, a tragic comedy or a Shakespearian drama. As fans we have enabled aberrant behavior by buying tickets, memorabilia, and simply watching the games on TV. That may seem harsh but it is true.

Surprisingly, there is gambling in pro sport. I have seen players in several sports think nothing of dropping $50,000 in a card game or $100,000 in a golf game with their friends. Drugs? Come on! We keep demanding more and more and there is only so much that the body can give. I really wonder if it would be better to open the whole thing up and recognize it for what it is. I love true sport, not this poor imitation we have.

The Athletic Development Process

Ultimately, I think we should all remember that the athletic development process is not something we do to the athlete, it is something we do with the athlete. Our job as professionals in athletic development is to help develop the most complete athlete we possibly can and to put that athlete into the competitive arena confident in their preparation so they can express their movement dynamics and ability to compete without reservation. There is definitely science to all of this and that cannot be rejected or denied.

But I also feel that the more I coach, the more I recognize the beauty and the wisdom of the body and the subsequent movements that the body is capable of performing. I'm sure if all of us would look at what we've done over the years, we would recognize that a lot of times—under the guise of coaching and direction—we've really created robots with a paint-by-numbers approach rather than provided our athletes with an empty canvas and a rich palate of colors to eventually paint a beautiful painting. That painting is their performance. It allows them the expression of their movement abilities to the optimum. This is all a very creative process. I truly believe that the current research in skill acquisition and coordination dynamics is telling us that what we have to do is give the athlete movement problems to solve, with the recognition and the understanding that a lot of times there are no correct answers. The athlete determines the correct answer.

And as we start this magical journey called athletic development, I think what we need to do is, first of all, understand the physical competencies necessary to achieve performance in the competitive arena. Then give the athletes the physical literacy to be able to strive in a healthy manner toward the achievement of performance in that competitive arena. We must recognize that it takes time. It is a long and circuitous path. The functional path is sometimes very well paved, and other times it is no more than a trail in the forest, so to speak.

Ultimately, recognize that the body is smart, and the body will find a way to solve movement problems. If you have any doubt about this, watch kids in free play in a natural environment. Watch athletic geniuses perform on the field and see how they adjust. Those adjustments happen too fast to take place on a cognitive level. We must recognize that, as athletic development professionals, we must teach them their athletic ABCs so that they can eventually produce a great novel of athletic performance.

This should never be about whether someone is right or wrong. My goal is to stimulate discussion and thought about why we do what we do, and when we do it. One-trick ponies are just that. We have to help develop the complete athlete. We can't afford to be one-trick ponies in training, because we are not one-trick ponies in the competitive arena. So we need to give the athlete a myriad of tools across a spectrum of demands that will enable them to achieve the highest level of athletic excellence relative to their potential. It is that simple.

Muscle Head Mentality

This is a passionate plea for sanity. If you are hanging your hat on an exercise, a machine or one concept, then what you are doing is creating athletes that are adapted. They adapt quickly to the exercise, be it the squat, clean, bench press, heavy sled pull, or whatever it is. But they are not adaptable. Can that adapted athlete then apply what they have done to become adapted to their movements in their sports? I would maintain that they can't.

We have made things like the Big Three an end unto themselves. We have made the power clean an end unto itself. We have lost sight of the big picture. The picture is to build a complete athlete who is completely adaptable to the demands of their sport with the training systematic, sequential and progressive.

I am seeing too many injuries coming from the "sheepwalking" mentality that forces athletes into methods and exercises that they are not ready for, or are inappropriate for their sport. If the training method cannot be adapted to the athlete then it is not a sound method! If the method can be adapted to the athlete, then it is sound and worth pursuing. This is another plea for the athletic development approach as opposed to the strength coach approach. Strength is only one component of athletic performance. There are many ways to acquire functional strength. Sure, you are never strong enough, as Mike Stone says, but that does not mean constantly seeking higher one-rep maximums. It really means understanding the spectrum approach to strength training that leads to applying various methods and forms of resistance relative to your stage of development, gender and sport.

With all the knowledge and understanding we have available to us as professionals (I use the term loosely), we are shooting ourselves in the foot. You folks out there who are university strength coaches, wake up! Sport coaches do not want their athletes going to the weight room because they never know what is going to come back out. I hear this all over the country. It certainly sends me a message—adapt or die.

The strength coach is the low man or women on the totem pole because they have allowed themselves to be, and because of the insular approach they have taken. You have created the Collegiate Strength and Conditioning Coaches Association (CSCCa) that feeds everyone's fantasy. Instead of going to CSCCa meetings, go to the soccer coaches convention, the swim coaches convention, the wrestling coaches convention, the volleyball coaches convention. You will learn more! Become a coach, not a weight room supervisor. I know soccer coaches, swim coaches, basketball coaches and track coaches who will not have their athletes go anywhere near the strength coach because he or she has their own agenda and will not listen to the input of the sport coach. The way I see it, if you are an athletic development coach then you are a resource to the sport coach. You can help them with program planning, recovery, nutrition and injury prevention. You can be an asset, not a liability.

Context, Context, Context

It is always all about context. Discussion on the squat brings this to the fore. It is not about the squat, or any exercise for that matter. It is the context in which the exercise is used and applied. That is my number one rule of thumb when designing training. I learned some cool exercises at the Level III coaching school, but I have to have a cooling off period to decide if they apply and when they apply to my system of training. Do not ever forget context.

Survive or Thrive: Is That the Question?

The other day I was watching a swimming workout. There were six or eight world-class swimmers and about twenty national-class swimmers. While watching the workout I was struck with the thought, how many of the swimmers are surviving the workout to come back and swim again for the next workout, and how many are thriving on the workout? The world-class group was OK but what about the others?

I think this is a fair question to ask when you have group training. I am always concerned about how the individual is going to react in a group training situation. I know I have that problem. Everyday I work with volleyball, and in the summer I have had up to 40 girls by myself, and someone or something will always fall between the cracks. Ideally, I would like to see everyone thrive on the workout and achieve positive adaptations but that is easier said than done. Addressing individual needs in a group context is always important, but difficult.

Words Into Images, Images Into Action

Here are three words that I feel should be eliminated from the lexicon of training. If you eliminate something then you should replace it with something better. In this case, I have carefully selected terms that more accurately describe the ultimate desired action. I was taught a long time ago that words create images in the mind, and that those images are then transferred into action. Therefore, we should be exacting and accurate in the words we select.

> *Strength and Conditioning.* Replace it with *athletic development*. This creates an image of athleticism and a blending of all components of performance, not just two components.

> *Periodization.* Replace it with *planned performance training*, because it is about timing of the development of the components of training and the subsequent adaptation to those components.

> *Prehab.* Replace it with *remedial*. Every athlete needs certain remedial work to prevent injury and to correct certain deficiencies. That work is remedial because it precedes more complex work to follow.

Can't or Won't

When an athlete says they cannot do something, that is very final. They can't do it. When they say they won't do it, that implies a choice. They can do it, but they have chosen not to do it at this time. I try to educate athletes and coaches on the distinction. I think it is an important distinction that we should all understand.

Finding Ideas

You must be constantly on the hunt for ideas and concepts that will make you better. To get ideas you must go outside your field, and broaden your interests. Read everything you can. Leave no stone unturned. Talk to coaches in a variety of sports. I am learning a ton each day from the volleyball coach I am working with. His drills are creative and purposeful. Read blogs in other fields. Diversify. Be a generalist. The pursuit of excellence is an ongoing process that has its own rewards.

Is Periodization Dead?

This was one of the questions asked at a presentation I gave to athletic and swim coaches at the University of Queensland. It is an important question. Periodization as it has been commonly taught by Bompa et al., is dead. That neat, defined world of general preparation, special preparation, competition and transition does not exist any more. Contemporary reality is that of an extended competitive season without well-defined, long periods of general preparation.

We must recognize that planning is still the cornerstone of all training, but we must not be bound by antiquated concepts that are derived from former Eastern Bloc nations that had strict control of their competitive schedule and total control of the athletes' lives. Traditional periodization also fails to adequately address the planning and preparation for team sports. We build upon principles of adaptation and current research to build plans that are realistic in our cultural and competitive milieu. Recognize that thorough and complete planning is a must. Please do not misinterpret what I am saying. We must be careful that we are not sleep walking and blindly following methodology that is outdated. There is a new reality that we must prepare for.

The Core

The term *core* is, as I suspected, a new term in the lexicon of training, therapy and medicine. Despite its popular use, no one has done a really good job of defining it from a scientific standpoint. It probably is not a big issue, but I am concerned when words begin to appear in peer-reviewed journals that have no accurate definition.

Essentially, right now it is a concept without specific definition. In an article titled, "Muscular Balance, Core Stability, and Injury Prevention for Middle and Long Distance Runners" by Michael Fredericson, M.D., and Tammara Moore, P.T., in *Physical Medicine Rehabilitation Clinics North America*, volume 16 pp. 669-689, they begin by stating the following:

> *Martial artists long have recognized the importance of a well developed core musculature. One of the main differences between a novice practitioner and a black belt is the black belt's development and use of his core (called "center" or "Ki") to produce balanced, powerful, and explosive movements.*

Later in the article, they go on to describe the core as follows:

> *In essence, the core can be viewed as a box with the abdominals in the front, paraspinals and gluteals in the back, the diaphragm as the roof, and the pelvic floor and hip girdle musculature as the bottom. Within this box are 29 pairs of muscles that help to stabilize the spine, pelvis, and kinetic chain during functional movements.*

This is actually a good start to a more accurate definition. It is very close to what Gajda and Dominguez published in 1983, in which they also included the thoracic and cervical spine.

The Choice: Adapted or Adaptable

My colleague, Steve Myrland, came up with the idea about the body being adapted or adaptable in response to training. It is a brilliant concept that demands a bit of explanation. Too much of what I see in training today results in bodies that are simply adapted to the specific type of work imposed upon them. Performance demands bodies that are adaptable to the demands of the sport. That is a much broader connotation that demands attention to the big picture.

It seems to me in designing and implementing a training program, the ultimate goal is to have a program that results in bodies that are completely adaptable. Adapted bodies are more prone to injury and will reach their performance limitations sooner. An adaptable body is the result of multifaceted training that covers a spectrum of activities designed to prepare the body for all aspects of the sport. The adaptable athlete will have few limitations. Biased one-sided training results in adapted bodies; multifaceted training results in adaptable bodies. What kind of body are you producing?

Lake Wobegon Effect

For those of you outside the United States, Lake Wobegon is a fictional town in Minnesota where humorist and social commentator Garrison Keillor supposedly was born. The famous tagline at the start of each vignette is, "Lake Wobegon, where the women are strong, the men are good looking, and all the children are above average," hence the identification of the Lake Wobegon Effect.

That is precisely where we are today. Everyone is not above average. Some people are good at certain skills and tasks, and not good at others. The mistaken notion has arisen that if we praise mediocre efforts they will magically become superior efforts. A mediocre effort is a mediocre effort no matter what words you use to describe it. We have raised a whole generation— in fact, several generations— with an inflated sense of self worth, because the adults have this mistaken notion that we can't allow kids to fail or to be average. How realistic is this? In the search for perfection we have created a dream world where there is no failure. Sports used to be the ultimate test. Now we give a trophy to everyone—how ridiculous. I was not always the first chosen. In fact many times I was the last chosen, and as a very late developer, any athletic ability remained well hidden for years. Did that deter me? No way, it drove me. I wanted to play with the big kids. I wanted to make varsity. Let's get realistic. By not allowing kids to face reality we are setting them up for bigger failures. We must praise effort that warrants praise, and correct poor effort. Lake Wobegon is fictional; life is real. Remember, without the "C" students where would the world be?

Change

Change is constant and it is uncomfortable. You can either fight change or embrace it and lead it. Kelvin Giles put it quite well when he said that coaches are change agents. That is what we do. Everyday we work to change and modify behavior in the form of fitness or skill, or even attitude. To lead change we must be comfortable with change. Leading change demands a willingness to at least consider new ideas and, if they are valid, implement them.

The Weight Room

Folks I will break it to you gently—the weight room is not the answer. For those of you who still think of yourselves as strength coaches I think it is time to reconsider what you are doing and how you are doing it. If the focus is on the weight room then the point of training the complete athlete is being missed. There are so many facets to athletic development that must be developed concurrently with strength that it is mind-boggling. In the past, I have received numerous e-mails with variations on the same theme: I turn my athletes over to the strength coach and the athletes get bigger and slower ... They are getting hurt in the weight room because everyone is doing the same program ... Everyone has to squat heavy (swimmers).

I have been on both sides of the fence here. I work with teams and schools to help them set up athletic development programs that are appropriate for their sport. Strength training is part of any sound athletic development program. Notice I said strength training. Strength training is an umbrella term. Under that umbrella comes a spectrum of activities and methods, from body weight gravitational load to heavy lifting to high speed, high force ballistic activities. What is appropriate for football where body mass and overcoming external resistance are key, is not appropriate for volleyball or swimming. One size does not fit all! Also, remember that strength training demands a different emphasis depending on the time of the competitive season. There are also different considerations for the female athlete; she must strength train more often and right through to the championship. (For example, Libby Lenton, the Australian swimmer, who won five gold medals in the 2007 World Swimming Championships, did her last strength training session on the Sunday with the World Championships beginning on Tuesday.)

I am once again making the case for athletic development instead of strength and conditioning. We must give the athletes the basic tools to thrive in their sports, not just survive. We must build athletic bodies that are adaptable to any athletic situation presented to them. Today, we are focusing on building bodies that are adapted to one environment and that environment does not often transfer to the field, court, pool and track.

I will end with an anecdote from my days with the White Sox. Charlie Hough, a knuckleball pitcher who pitched in the major leagues until his late-forties, used to call it the *wait room* where he used to sit on a bench smoking cigarettes while he waited to pitch. On the other days he used it to strength train in the weight room. He had a program that worked for him—he sought input from Steve Odgers and myself, and incorporated what would work for him.

Australian Institute of Sport (AIS)

My first visit to the AIS was in 1996. The AIS is located in Canberra, the capital of Australia. It is inland, about a three-hour drive from Sydney. It reminds me very much of the foothills of the Sierra Mountains in California. There have been significant changes in facilities; the library/information center has tripled in size. It is an unbelievable resource. Someday I want to go back and spend a week just doing research. They have every possible resource imaginable pertaining to sport. They have a new recovery center adjacent to a new 50-meter pool and a huge new weight room. They have a new department devoted entirely to studying skill acquisition. The biomechanics lab has been completely redone. There is a 30-meter-long force platform in the track as part of the lab. Just imagine what you could do with that. Most importantly, I think it is the people they have there. The facilities are impressive, but they have good people who are passionate and knowledgeable—there to serve the athlete.

What I Learned Down Under

1. It is about people, not facilities and equipment. The Australians have a culture that values sport and coaching.

2. Integration of sport science is part of the sporting culture. The input of the sport scientist is sought and valued.

3. Just like us, they have their problems. Sometimes they are

top heavy with administration. Government funding is both a blessing and a curse, at times.

4. Friendships through sport are long lasting and built on mutual respect.

5. They have a real desire to learn and improve. They look for the edge by seeking new knowledge. When you have a small population you must use all resources possible to develop talent.

6. The difference between coaching and personal training was reaffirmed.

7. There are no secrets. People were open and willing to share ideas and information.

8. Our American football could learn a tremendous amount from Rugby Union, Rugby League and Aussie Rules Football.

9. They no longer have required physical education in the schools. We both need it.

10. Recovery for them is much more scientific. It is based on the demands of the practice or the game.

QAS (Queensland Academy of Sport) Swim Squad

What an impressive group. Libby Lenton headlines the squad. She was the winner of five gold medals in the 2007 World Swimming Championships. She is also a multiple world-record holder. The coach is Stephan Widmer, another friend from my previous visit. When I met Stephan in 1999 he was the assistant coach, but obviously a coach on the rise.

We spent the afternoon talking about training, and exchanging ideas. It was refreshing to talk to a coach of this caliber who was willing to openly share ideas. We talked extensively about the dry land program and compared notes about what they do and what I have done with the Michigan women. It is a squad of men and women—nine swimmers total, so practice is not about crowd control. It is about quality work with quality attention on the athletes. Everything was done with a purpose. There is a huge emphasis on technique and learning how to swim fast. No garbage yardage here. There is a complete focus on excellence.

The detailed preparation was impressive. He uses a timed swim at 15 meters as a benchmark to ascertain where they are in terms of speed at all times. Libby Lenton was coming off a three-week break, and being a bit sick, she just worked on drills and getting the feel back for her stroke. Stephan works hard to build a sense of team within the squad.

The Overhead Myth Won't Go Away

A reader wrote the following:

> I have been working with a university women's volleyball team for some time now (approx. 5 yrs). I use a functional approach to their training and have had quite good success over the years. Recently, four of our players attended a National U21 camp where they stood out as being the fittest group there. As part of the camp they had sessions with the athletic therapy staff and strength and conditioning staff for more of an information session than actual training program administration. During the session with the strength and conditioning coaches, one of the coaches told them they should avoid at all cost overhead pressing. We do include both overhead pressing and pulling movements in our current program to allow for a good strength base when they are at the net blocking, etc., but we do not do any overhead work

that requires high velocity. None of it involves behind the head type work though. I would love to hear your comments regarding overhead pressing and/or pulling for overhead athletes such as volleyball, baseball, tennis, etc.

This ranks right in there with the not letting the knee go beyond the toe and the toe up (dorsiflexion) in sprinting. I use overhead movements all the time in all the sports you mentioned. I have used those movements for years. It is not that the overhead movement can be the problem, it is how you get overhead. Remember that the shoulder is connected to the hip, and the hip leads. In all those sports you mentioned the overhead movement is a direct performance factor, therefore it must be trained in a systematic manner. One key is that the overhead movements must correlate with what is happening in practice. I am careful not to add fatigue to fatigue. Remember, it is our job to prepare the athlete athletically so that the sport coach can optimize technique and skill. Old myths die hard!

The Knee Past the Toe: Here We Go!

Just about the time I thought the issue of the knee going past the toe was dead, it keeps rearing its ugly head. It is hard to believe that this is still an issue, considering what we understand about knee function. Approach this with an analytical mind. Start by observing movement. Observe the knee in work, play and games, and ask yourself the following questions:

Where does the knee go?
How does it get there?
How does it get back to where it started?

Observe how the ankle, knee and hip link and synchronize. All of these movements occur in hundredths to tenths of a second. You cannot consciously think about where the knee should go—it all happens too fast. It is all subcortical and reflexive, not planned and programmed. This demands that training progressively loads the knee in all the positions that could occur in the demands of the sport. Artificially restricting knee motion will not prevent knee injuries; in fact, you may be setting up the knee for injury.

Here is a simple mantra to guide your training involving the knee: Link and Sync—Don't Think.

Five Minds For The Future

I thoroughly enjoyed this book by Howard Gardner. For those of you who are not familiar with him, Gardner is a cognitive psychologist from Harvard who is credited with originating the theory of multiple intelligences in his book, *Frames of Mind*. In this book he defines the five minds that are necessary to thrive in our fast changing world:

The Disciplined Mind—Mastery of major schools of thought, the capability of applying oneself beyond formal education.

The Synthesizing Mind—Selecting key information from copious amounts of information.

The Creating Mind—Going beyond the boundaries of existing disciplines and asking new questions and offering new solutions.

The Respectful Mind—Recognizing differences in individuals and groups and learning to work with those differences.

The Ethical Mind—Striving toward good work and good citizenship.

Stretching and Warm-up

Stretching is not warm-up. I repeat, stretching is not warm-up. Several dynamic stretches should be part of warm-up. Those stretches should be placed in the latter third of warm-up when the body is warm. Also, group stretching is an almost complete waste of time. Stretching must fit each individual based on his or her needs. All of that being said go watch warm-up in MLB or the NBA and you will see millions of dollars of bodies wallowing around on the ground doing static stretching at the start of warm-up. Usually that takes half to two-thirds of the whole warm-up. Stretching has a place, but it is not warm-up.

Happy Days are Here Again!

Why are we seeing some of the things we see today, that we have never seen before? The younger generation is not taught the basics of movement. Sure, your generation knows a lot; that is great, but can that knowledge be applied? I have seen way too many younger coaches who know a lot but do not have the common sense to come out of the rain. Don't deny the past, learn from it—both the good and the bad. I had more terrible coaches than good coaches in the good old days. They have been my inspiration all my life. I vowed at an early age to never be like them. So, in summary, everything old is not necessarily good, nor is everything new the best, either; it is a good combination of experience and knowledge.

Interesting Conversation

The wedding of my daughter's best friend was really fun. At the reception dinner there was a lady sitting next to my wife who had just retired after 30 years of being a middle school PE

FOLLOWING THE FUNCTIONAL PATH

teacher here in Sarasota. This lady really got it. She graduated from Ball State when there was a curriculum to prepare teachers how to teach. She said she was appalled at the young teachers coming out of school today. She said they know the sport they played, but have no idea how to teach skill or organize a class for effective teaching. We both agreed that in this case it would be good to turn back the clock and teach PE teachers how to teach.

Playing the Game

How important is it to have played the game in order to coach? I think it depends on whether you are an athletic development coach or an actual sport coach. If you are a sport coach, to have some exposure to the game as a player at some level is important. With professional baseball the pedigree they often look for is someone who has played Major League Baseball. This results in little creativity or innovation. I think Bill Belichick is the coach he is because he did not play pro football. From a conditioning coach's perspective, I really do not think it is necessary; in fact, it is an advantage to have not played the game. There is less bias and preconceived notions, hence more objectivity.

Certification: Educational or Entrepreneurial?

I am all for education and knowledge. I feel even more strongly than I ever have that more certification does not mean more knowledge. In fact, there are so many certifications now that it is confusing. Do we have more knowledge because of these certifications or do we have more information being passed around as knowledge? How many letters can you have after your name before they start becoming insignificant? When I see someone 20-something with more than one degree and one certification after their name, I get suspicious. Have they been gathering information or seeking knowledge? Why do you have to be certified in an exercise technique or a piece of equipment? If your knowledge is based on sport science, and grounded in a sound philosophy, why do you need it? A method or a piece of equipment must be placed in context. Rather than add credibility, it takes away credibility.

The newest one I just saw last night is that you can become a core pole master trainer. What on earth is a core pole and do you need to be a master trainer to use it? Here is another good one—online training expert. Wow, is that impressive. You can join the Personal Trainer Business Alliance. They even have a competency and ethics expert on board! Let's get real here and take a stand as professionals. Everyone must make a living, but are we duping the public by falsely inflating the knowledge base of these various certifications? Perhaps the competency and ethics expert should take a look at this. By the way, PT means physical therapist not personal trainer. There is a difference.

We do not need more certifications. That is not the solution to define this field. At the last count, there are over 300 certifications in this field. Will another certification help define the field or add more confusion? More letters are not the answer! We must find a way to professionalize what we do, and have standards that are universally accepted. There must be standards of proficiency. How about experience and professional competence?

I do believe in certification. I believe in certification with substance. By substance I mean programs that require apprenticeships with a recognized professional in the field. It should entail a significant hands-on educational component. For example, a week-long course that has a blend of theoretical and practical information would be useful. It has to be much more than a paper-and-pencil test or an online video review. There must be a project that shows original thinking and a depth of knowledge. In short, it should be rigorous so that it has substance, so that potential employers have a better idea of what they are getting. It should have levels that reflect the hierarchy of knowledge and time served—experience, which just reflects sound pedagogy. No one should be grandfathered into a program. There is much more, but I think that should give you an idea of where I am coming from.

Over the years, beginning in the late '60s, I have studied coaching education programs in a wide variety of sports all over the world. When we started the USA Track and Field Coaching Education Program in 1983 the goal was to raise the standard of coaching. We leaned heavily on the Canadian, Australian, and British models already in existence for guidance. The program continues today. It is a sound program. In many ways it is one of the best programs available in the United States today. Does it have holes and faults? Of course. It is run entirely by volunteers. In other countries the coaching education schemes are run by paid professionals. We need to go this route with athletic development or there will always be confusion. My intent is to get people to think, and to raise the standard of coaching.

The Leg Circuit

Body Weight Squat x 20 reps
Body Weight Lunge x 20 reps (10 each leg)
Body Weight Step-up x 20 reps (10 each leg)
Jump Squat x 10

The order of the exercises is important. I arrived at the order by trial and error. This order allows the exercises to be done with a degree of quality. Rate of work is also crucial. The goal is one rep per second, as this really stresses the fast eccentric muscle action, which is a key element in body weight lower-extremity exercise. Last, but not least, remember context—this is one part of a detailed long-term progression. The leg circuit is not an end unto itself. It will give you a real burn, but that is not what it is about. It is about foundational strength to provide a work capacity of power endurance to build upon.

The Secret

After all this thinking and writing about coaching and defining a field I decided to call Joe Vigil. I realized I had not spoken to him in a while and wanted to see how he was doing. Man, did that call get me fired up! Joe has to be one of the most amazing and inspiring individuals I have ever met. Joe is in his mid- to late-70s but you would never know it. He is just as fired up as when I first met him 25 years ago. The more I spoke to him, the more I realized that he knows the secret. The secret is passion. He has passion for coaching, learning and teaching that rates a 12.5 on a 10.0 scale. He gets up every morning at 5:00 A.M. to do one hour of reading for professional advancement. This is a guy with a Ph.D. and several master's degrees. He has forgotten more than most of us know and he is reading for professional advancement.

Passion—that is the answer; it is the secret. People like Joe are a prized resource. He has never gotten the respect and adulation he deserves. I know I would not be anywhere that I am today without Joe Vigil's help and advice.

The formula is KNOWLEDGE + INTEGRITY + PASSION.

What is Coaching?

Are coaching and personal training different? Yes. Training someone for a short period of time is not the same as the commitment to work with an athlete's training for a year or a career, and having to manage that training with all that comes with it. Coaching deals with all the variables. You can't pop in and pop out on an hourly basis and be a coach.

Importance of History

Ken Burns, the documentary filmmaker, said the following when delivering the commencement address at Georgetown University in 2006: "As you pursue your goals in life, that is to say your future, pursue your past. Let it be your guide. Insist on having a past and then you will have a future."

Do not descend too deeply into specialism in your work. Educate all your parts. You will be healthier. Replace cynicism with its old-fashioned antidote, skepticism.

If you do not know where you have been, how can you possibly know where you are and where you are going?"

How many of you have read the works of Doc Councilman? How about John Bunn's book or the numerous books that Ken Doherty wrote? Heed the advice of Ken Burns: Learn about the past to make your present and future more meaningful.

Analytics

Do you know why the things you are doing in training work or do not work? Are you just following your intuition or some artificial model that you fit your athletes into? I just finished an interesting book published by Harvard Business School Press called *Competing on Analytics: The New Science of Winning*, by Thomas Davenport and Jeanne Harris. This really got me thinking that what is being done in the business sector must be done in coaching. There are too many exorbitant claims without any substance. Also, we need to be able to repeat what we do. How can you repeat what works if you do not know why it worked or if it really does work?

"Just the Facts"

One of my favorite television programs growing up was Dragnet. The star of the program was Sergeant Joe Friday of the LAPD. His famous line was, "Just the facts" when he was interrogating a witness. Little did I know how right-on Sergeant Friday was. Cut out the hype, the marketing and the misinformation. Cut to the chase. What works? Why does it work? Is it repeatable? Can you teach it? What is necessary to achieve mastery? Just the facts!

Innovation/Change

Are innovation and change synonymous? The spirit is what is important—the willingness to plough new ground and go where no one else has dared to venture before. Put it out there. Do what works; prove the way later. Whatever you do should be guided by principles.

Pedigree

I am definitely not a betting man, but if I were to bet on the horses I would thoroughly investigate a horse's pedigree before I bet on that horse. I think it is the same in coaching and teaching. Pedigree and lineage mean a lot. Who were your mentors? Who did you learn from? You can't choose your parents, but you can choose your mentors; that will determine your pedigree. More letters after your name do not improve your pedigree. Gain knowledge and experience to improve your pedigree, then you will be a winner. Remember Seabiscuit did not have the pedigree, but that horse had people who believed in him and sought out the knowledge to make him better. If they had listened to conventional wisdom, Seabiscuit would not have been a winner. Create your own pedigree.

Some Random Thoughts

Here are some things I have been thinking about:

• Kids should play and adults should train.

• Plyometrics are okay for kids as long as there are no adults telling them what to do. Jumping, hopping and bounding are natural. Let them play at it.
• Same with strength training for kids. Let them climb, pull and push; just don't organize and see how much they can lift. In fact do not let them in the weight room—give them rocks, trees, tires and medicine balls and go for it!

• Olympic-style weight lifters are good athletes who are skilled in a very narrow set of skills. They get very explosive, but if that explosiveness always transfers why don't we see eight weight lifters line up for the final of the 100 meters?

• Have you ever seen a world-class 5,000-meter runner run a fast 1,000 meters with a training flat on one foot and a spike on the other foot? I have! Talk about crazy stuff!

• Typical advice—Don't work too hard because you might get hurt. Then you get hurt because you did not work hard enough.

• Michael Phelps, the Olympic swimmer, attributed his recent success to weight training and plyometrics. Now we will see every age group swimmer in the U.S. weight training and doing plyometrics, with no idea of how to start, how to progress, and in what context they were done.

• Training is not an all-you-can-eat buffet. It is a gourmet meal carefully prepared so all the ingredients are planned and blended into a fine dining experience.

Daisuke Matsuzaka: Change Agent?

The other day, I met two of my friends from my White Sox days for lunch. They both now work for the Houston Astros. Dewey Robinson is the Pitching Development Coordinator and Jaime Garcia is his assistant. They were talking about an article in *Sports Illustrated* concerning the Japanese pitcher, Daisuke Matsuzaka, who is now pitching for the Boston Red Sox. When I got home from a workout I read the article.

It was a breath of fresh air to me. Matsuzaka's training habits and his ability to achieve high pitch counts in games, and then do a high volume of throwing between starts, has caused quite a stir in the closed, conservative world of baseball. If you get a chance, read the article in the March 26, 2007 Baseball Preview issue of *Sports Illustrated*.

The following are my comments stimulated by the article and reflecting my personal experience as Director of Conditioning for the Chicago White Sox for nine years and as Director of Athletic Development for the New York Mets for eight months.

Will Matsuzaka's training habits and approach to pitching change the American approach? I hope so, because change is needed. We have put the pitcher on a pedestal and forgotten to train him, and then marvel at the extent and severity of the injuries that continue to occur. In reaction to the injuries, we have them throw less. We must train them to tolerate the demands of pitching. We must recognize the demands of pitching as a ballistic explosive activity, and train for those demands. Matsuzaka also does not ice after he throws. I really do not know why that is so revolutionary. We instituted that as a policy in the minor leagues with the White Sox in 1989. I thoroughly researched the physiology of icing then and have continued to follow the research, and there is not a physiological reason to ice a healthy shoulder or elbow. In fact, it may be counterproductive. I am glad he is getting publicity for that because maybe it will force people to re-evaluate icing.

As far as the amount of throwing he does in the bullpen and in long toss, it certainly does not seem unreasonable to me for someone who has progressed to that level. The key here is to progress to that level. Our young players pitch too much and do not throw enough. They need to condition to throw and then throw to condition. Throw anything when they are in their developmental stages—softballs, football, rocks, or just play throwing games where they have to use different angles and positions of the body. That will prepare them to pitch. Instead, we train them in a phone booth. We teach them a narrow range of throwing skills called pitching mechanics and lock them into that movement repetitively, and then wonder why they get sore and hurt. In essence, we are cloning pitchers so they all look alike. There is no model. Let them find their pattern and then condition them to withstand the forces.

Throw away the radar gun! The obsession with velocity is the root of all evil. Everyone in the game preaches location and control and the ability to throw strikes, but then judges the pitcher on velocity. No one really knew how hard Bob Feller or Sandy Koufax threw, and did it matter?

Forget the argument that a pitcher has only so many pitches in him—that is absurd. The fact that doctors have said this has lent it credibility, but there is no science behind this. That reminds me of the argument before Roger Bannister broke the four-minute barrier in the mile, that there are only so many heartbeats, so don't use them up by training hard!

Here are five rules for training the pitcher:

1. Build the pitcher from the ground up. You can't launch a cannon from a canoe; build strong legs.

2. Train toenails to fingernails—train all the links in the chain to produce and reduce force.

3. Train for power and explosiveness, not endurance.

4. Train the core as a relay center. The trunk positions the arms and transfers force from the legs.

5. Focus on the big picture—recognize that the shoulder and elbow are the last links in the kinetic chain.

Recognize also that you have many "experts" weighing in on this argument who have no background in sport science or training. They have never had to produce by keeping a pitcher healthy and developing a young pitcher. You can look at all the stats you want, but you must know the individual pitcher, understand the biomechanics, and have a principle-based program.

In many respects this comes back to physical education. Get them moving and playing. Put the softball throw back into the President's Fitness Test, and you will see throwing improve.

I sincerely hope that Matsuzaka has success because it may force the sport to take a hard look at training. Knowing baseball, and the conservative nature of the game, I really doubt that any change will occur even if he wins 20 games. Baseball is a game defined by failure. Secretly, you can bet that everyone in the game is wishing he will fail so that they can keep doing what they have always done—spit, scratch and chew.

More Thoughts on Words

Words create images and images create action. Here are some common misinterpretations of words in the context of training:

Workout = Weight Room
Warm-up = Stretching
Conditioning = Distance Running
Fitness = Wind Sprints
Basics = Boring

Fat, Fit or What?

Fat or fit: Does that have to be the choice? An article in
USA Today had a front-page story on the sad state of the recruits
entering the military. One-third of the 18-year olds who applied for
service in all branches of the military were overweight. Between
1996 and 2006 the applicants considered obese doubled to six
percent. In speaking with people who have worked with army
recruits they report the rate of stress fractures in recruits as high as
50 percent.

Should we be alarmed? Yes, we should. We do not have to worry
about terrorist attacks; if they wait a few years we will just eat
ourselves into oblivion! This is a huge problem (no pun intended)
that permeates all levels of society. Unfortunately, there are no
simple solutions.

Ironically, the poor state of fitness of military recruits before WWII
was considered a problem. It was recognized as a problem and there
were mechanisms in place to deal with it. The top experts in physical
education were gathered and the physical education curriculums
were revised to better prepare the youth for the war on the horizon.

We certainly need a national initiative of concerned people to
reverse this alarming trend. Unfortunately, we are not teaching
physical education as a discipline in the colleges and universities
because it is not a requirement in the secondary and elementary
schools. There are no jobs, so we are not training the teachers who
can go out and lead. The curriculums that are in place in the schools

leave much to be desired. The so-called *new* PE does not get the job done. It appears the goal of the *new* PE is to keep the kids happy and not stress them. We must step back and be realistic.

In the same vain, Charlie Crist, then-Governor of Florida, proposed that Florida institute a mandatory 30 minutes of physical education a day. That is fine, but how will it be implemented? Who will teach it? That is the clincher. A clue was the advisory board that he named. It contained all professional athletes, but not one educator. We do not need politicians involved in this. We need educators who understand what must be done. PE is an integral part of the educational process. Studies have consistently shown that children who move and participate in vigorous activities do better in school and have fewer behavioral issues in the classroom. We need to start a grassroots revolution among people who are concerned. It must be done. Talk is cheap. We need a call to action to get kids fit for life!

Some way, somehow, we must change the patterns of behavior and get people to rethink their approach to fitness. I am convinced that this revolution must be led by leaders in individual communities. I am really not sure how to go about this; that is why I am throwing out this idea. There are certainly bright, innovative people out there who can get this going. Maybe we need to think of this like a virus—start small in your neighborhood and let it spread. One thing that I am convinced of, is that throwing more money at the problem without a plan will have minimal impact.

Appearances Can Fool You

I received this interesting question from a reader recently:

While vacationing in Florida for spring break, I had a chance to observe minor league teams working out. What caught my attention was the conversation between a player and one of the strength coach/trainers. The trainer was commenting to one of the players, who was running, that they were lazy and did not know how to train; and stated, "I can outrun anyone in this camp." By looking between the two, the trainer who has this Adonis physique and the portly pitcher/player, my buddy said, "Twenty bucks... the trainer will outrun this guy." To make the story short, not only did the portly player outrun the Adonis physique strength coach, the player embarrassed the whole strength staff. Vern, can you explain to me why a portly player outran a physically fit strength professional?

This is an interesting story that must be answered on two levels. First, it is probably not advisable to challenge athletes you are working with to a competition. It is a no-win situation. If you beat them, what does that prove? If you do not, then you lose their respect. Neither alternative is acceptable. Also, they are professional athletes for a reason; you are not. Demonstrate the activity, don't challenge their ability to do the skill. Teach them how to do it.

The second level to the answer is to never judge a book by its cover. Looking buff and being fit are two different things. Appearance is certainly deceiving. As coaches, sometimes we are quick to judge by appearances. The real question is, what are you fit for? Also, how do you measure fitness? Is max VO2 important for baseball, as a team doctor once told me? Bottom line is to know the game you are preparing for; the training you do should be appropriate for the sport you are training for. Pitching is a good example. Why do pitchers have to do the amount of running they do? It certainly does not reflect the demands of their activity, which is a series of very explosive bursts lasting less than two seconds with 25-to-30 seconds recovery. Also a pitcher does not have to look like Adonis to pitch effectively. Remember: Force = Mass x Acceleration. Nobody ever said that the mass had to be all muscle. It is nice to see a pitcher who looks good in a uniform, but the ultimate measure is to be able to perform and stay healthy.

American Football

I do very little with American football—this was a conscious choice when I quit playing football a long time ago. But that does not mean that I have not closely observed the training scene for the past 45 years. Over the years, I have worked with some individual players at all levels of the game, and have consulted with some coaches who were willing to innovate. I find American football quite stifling and uncreative both in regards to tactic and strategy, and conditioning. I know I have to be careful about painting with too broad a brush, but the monkey-see, monkey-do syndrome is all pervasive. One person started flipping tires and won a few games, then everybody started to flip tires. I've no idea where and how it fits into the big picture, but because it is hard and sometimes they throw up when they are doing it, it has to be good—or so they think. This is indicative of the trickle-down effect that starts at the top and ends up in the youth leagues. There is little regard for development level and sound progressions. The emphasis is on getting big and getting strong. Freshmen should not be doing the same program as seniors, whether at the high school or the collegiate level. Positions should be trained differently based on the demands of the position.

I think a good way to look at it is to contrast American football with Rugby Union and Rugby League. Both play very demanding schedules, in some more so than American football. For example, in the English Premier League they play from September through May with international games thrown in. There is no situational substation, so a high level of fitness is required. They are collision sports, so you must have bulk for padding and strength to move people. I have seen, as I am exposed more to rugby, that they are much more progressive and innovative than American football. They are doing things that American football has never thought of.

I see some of the things that my colleague Dean Benton is doing with the Brisbane Broncos and I am amazed. I can't help but think what an edge those things would give an American football team it they would adopt them. The New Zealand All Blacks are doing training monitoring that is state of the art. What Kelvin Giles is doing with the Australian Rugby Union Development Squad (14 to 17 in residence), is great stuff that takes into consideration proper progressions, and growth and development. What I see in the rugby situations is sport science-based training coupled with good coaching and player development models.

American football needs to wake up and learn that there is a big world out there that they can learn from. There is enormous room for innovation that would significantly improve athleticism and reduce injuries. Remember, it is tough to solve a problem by going to those who created it. Happy combine training!

Formula for Failure II

I did not write the following—a very good friend wrote it. It really does not matter which sport it refers to, because it could be any sport. I have seen this so may times myself. The moral of this story, is that we need to stop passing around mythology and keep trying to define what we do from as scientific a viewpoint as possible. Unfortunately, many times coaching is ahead of science. That means that, as coaches, we try to be as scientific as possible. There is a method to the madness. We also need to beware of pseudo-science and false claims, which are prevalent because of the Internet and the speed of communication possible today. Remember, search for knowledge not information!

This is based on a true story, but the sport and the names have been hidden to protect the innocent.

Once upon a time, there was a young athlete in an individual sport, trying his best to excel. He kept making an error though, which held him back. Not understanding what was actually happening, he made a change in his approach that appeared to solve his particular problem.

Because this change worked for him, he decided to write an article on this and it became popular in the U.S....but not in Europe. In fact, thousands of words were later written on this change...and for most U.S. coaches, hey, this is the gospel. It is the gospel called "hearsay".

Even before this athlete made this personal adjustment in technique, biomechanists were studying the event, frame by frame. They used force plates, fancy cameras, super software programs, and they came to a conclusion the young athlete couldn't understand. The science showed that whatever the young athlete did was sort of an aberration. "Here, look at all of these elite athletes. The pattern clearly shows that doing exactly the opposite of what you did, will produce WR results." Funny... you know that the biomechanists were right! They came from various countries, but their studies all agree. In the U.S., maybe because of funding, no biomechanists commented on this particular move.

I can tell you...the sport wasn't golf or tennis, because you readers would all know there are tons written on those sports.

Meanwhile, WR's were set by non-Americans, Olympics were won...and, the Americans had mustard on their shirts, not medals. (The Americans didn't make the finals, so they ate hot dogs instead!) Wouldn't you think that the American coaches would start to think: HEY, maybe this move we do only in the U.S. is WRONG!! You would think. Sadly, the situation is that most of the coaches believe the hearsay, rather than the science.

The moral of the story is this: Do your homework. Go to the top experts in your field, even if they are overseas! Look for references to back up statements. Try to be as scientific as possible.

Experience Does Matter

I have read many articles and interviews with performance directors at various training centers commenting on training. Not one of them was over 30. I do not think you have to be an old man or woman to direct a program or to be an expert, but experience does matter. I was a young Turk once, who knew everything and was not afraid to tell anyone who would listen, and some who would not listen, what I knew. I was sure I knew everything. I am convinced now that taking that stance was a real impairment to my learning. How can you learn when you know everything?

There is a real value to knowing what you don't know. Sometimes it is more important than knowing what you do know. In today's fast-paced world of instant results and quick fixes it is easy to get caught up in hype and promotion. Everyday as I coach, I see and do things now that I learned through experience. There's no book or class to prepare you for the reality of day-to-day coaching. All of you who are younger in your careers, seek out mentors who have been doing this for a while and have achieved success. I know how helpful Joe Vigil has been to me, and continues to be to this day. Hang out with people who challenge you and make you better. One thing Joe said to me was to gain experiences, not have the same experience over and over. Learn from failure. We all fail. Those who ultimately are successful are those who learn from their failures and do not repeat them.

Experience is what a person does with what they know. It is like Joe Vigil says, you can be coaching 30 years and have one experience 30 times or you can have 30 experiences. To me it is all about the latter. One thing I do know for certain now, is that things are sure a lot clearer to me looking back over the years and reviewing past successes and failures, in order to not repeat the failures and to build upon the successful experiences. I know now that I would not have been ready after five or ten years to assume some of the positions I see people in today. It probably reflects a different era.

In 1979, I was one of four finalists for the position of head track and field coach at Stanford University. I was disappointed that I did not get the job, but when I look back I was not ready for the job. I had only been coaching for ten years and definitely needed many more experiences and some failures to humble me. *Sports Illustrated* (March 19, 2007) had a superb article about the 1964 UCLA basketball team, John Wooden's first NCAA championship team. The team had no starter over 6'5"! I recommend that everyone interested in coaching and excellence read it. Several points in the article underscore the importance of experience. One of his guiding principles was, "It's what you learn after you know it all that counts." This man is considered one of the greatest coaches of all time. When he speaks, I listen. I just wish I had listened more when I was younger.

The Athletically Gifted

Reading the article, "The Effort Effect," about the work of Stanford psychologist Carol Dweck in Stanford's alumni magazine, got me thinking. She has been doing research to determine why some people achieve their potential and others fall by the wayside. This certainly hit home with me. It caused me to reflect on those I have seen who did not make it and those who did.

In the course of my coaching career I have been fortunate to see two athletes start at the developmental level and progress to be the best in the world. I have been reflecting quite a bit on this lately as I see the inordinate amount of emphasis put on finding and identifying the athletically gifted. I realize that the conditions that nurtured these youngsters were in a different era and under a different set of circumstances. One of the two individuals I am referring to is Terry

Schroeder, who went on to be acknowledged as the best water polo player in the world and is considered one of the all time greats in the sport. He is now a chiropractor and the water polo coach at Pepperdine University. I was fortunate to have Terry in an eighth-grade PE class in 1970-71.

The second individual is Karch Kiraly, who is considered one of the greatest volleyball players ever—both indoors and on the beach. He was a student at Santa Barbara High School when I coached there. I did not have much direct contact with him, but was able to observe and follow his development.

These two men developed into the best in their respective sports and among the best ever. Why? I have often thought about that and about what is different today. I often wonder, if they were growing up today, would they have achieved the status they've attained? They were not anointed at a young age, although Karch did receive some attention for his prowess on the beach, playing against older players. Both were humble and worked hard to achieve their success. Schroeder did not even start playing water polo until he was a sophomore in high school. He was a good age group swimmer, a good football player, a good basketball player and a good baseball player, but certainly not a prodigy in any of those sports. He did not mature early, but because of his multi-sport background he was very coordinated and learned skills rapidly. He was also very intelligent.

Karch was a prodigy. His dad had been a good volleyball player in Hungary and started him playing very young. I remember seeing him as a five-year old on the beach and being taken aback by his skills. He never let that go to his head. To my knowledge, he did not play other sports, although I did try to persuade him to go out for track. He worked hard and smart. He was also very intelligent, majoring in pre-med at UCLA. I do know that both of them had physical education daily throughout their school years. I do not know if that made a huge difference, but it had to have had some benefit.

As I reflect on this, there are many lessons to be learned from these two athletes' ultimate success on the world stage. They seemed to be able to maintain a perspective as the spotlight began to shine on them. They had good fundamental movement skills that served as a base for their specific sport skills. They played a lot—I emphasize play! They were very intelligent. They had parents who cared, but did not seem overbearing. They were goal-achievement oriented. I am not sure their paths could be replicated in today's world of early specialization and media hype.

PTs and ATCs

In the past I have written about physical therapists and here is one comment I received:

> "Would love to hear more about your experience at GLATA (Great Lakes Athletic Trainers' Association), and your thoughts/ opinions of this, based on your interaction with both athletic trainers and physical therapists."

The program for the GLATA convention was impressive. Looking at the program you would have to say that the profession of athletic training has come a long way. They certainly have professionalized themselves over the years. Up to a point, I think the field of strength and conditioning could learn some things from the athletic trainers and their governing body, the NATA (National Athletic Trainers' Association).

That being said, I think over the past couple of years athletic trainers have been going down a one-way street in the wrong direction. They are trying to be what they are not, and probably were not intended to be. They are not physical therapists. As I understand it, their job is to provide primary care in an athletic and clinical setting. I understand that in many situations, because a need arises, they must condition and rehab the athlete, but that is not their primary job. I have the utmost respect for ATCs and the role they play in keeping

FOLLOWING THE FUNCTIONAL PATH

athletes healthy and performing. Sometimes it is too easy to get caught up in trying to be something that we do not need to be.

I know I am oversimplifying this issue, but that is my point of view as a coach and one who has hired ATCs and been in charge of them in a professional setting. It is my understanding that the hours in the training, that were once a requirement, have been modified. That is a shame, if that is true. I always felt that the practical experience in the training room gave the beginning trainer an advantage coming out of school. That is unlike the strength and conditioning coach who only has to pass a paper-and-pencil test. I hope the old guard in the training profession will stop and be the voice of reason on all of this.

Let it Happen

First you learn to play, and then you forget what you learned and just play! This is a paraphrase of what I heard a jazz musician say in an interview on NPR (National Public Radio). When I heard it, I could not help but think of this in the context of athletic skills. Learn it, then drill it and don't think—let it happen! Let the instincts and the subcortical responses take over. It was Charlie Parker who said: "Master your instrument. Master the music. And then forget all that bull___ and just play."

The Weight Room

Recently, I heard a conversation between two coaches that went something like this: "Have you looked at the record board lately?" The other coach says, "No." The first coach says, "They are getting so strong I can't believe it!" He goes on to say how much better they will be because they are so much stronger. I had to bite my tongue and not say anything. This group of athletes the coach was talking about had to be one of the most unathletic groups I have seen. They were unfit and sloppy looking. I wanted to ask if they could move. I would bet that although these players were putting up some pretty good numbers in the weight room, that they would struggle to handle their own body weight in push-ups, pull-ups, lunges, and crawling—in short, any movements that forced them to control their bodies through three planes of movement. I am not opposed to weight training. A football player who does not weight train will not survive on the field because they need to add mass for protection and they must move their opponents. I do, however, think that most football strength coaches do not get it! If the strength developed in the weight room cannot be applied on the field, then it is not useful strength.

This may seem contradictory but it is not. It is really about proper program planning. It still goes back to one of the fundamental Functional Path Principles—body weight before external resistance. In other words, prepare for the heavy lifting. Make sure the ligaments and tendons surrounding the joints are prepared, and that a strong muscular corset around the core is developed. This takes time, but when they finally do make the heavy lift, they will be able to lift more weight safely and apply that strength to the field. Movement ability must be developed in parallel to the strength development. It is not an either/or proposition. The weight room is only one part of a much bigger picture.

Piece by Piece

Building the complete athlete takes time, and a clear vision of the big picture. Once that vision is established then you can look at the pieces, or components, of the training. The analogy of assembling a jigsaw puzzle is a good one. When you take the puzzle out of the box there are hundreds of pieces on the table in a completely random order. The reference is the picture of the completed puzzle on the cover of the box. Just like training, you cannot force the pieces into places where they do not belong. You know where the pieces fit by constantly referencing the completed picture. The mistake too many people make in training the athlete, is trying to force pieces to fit where they do not belong. Part of the cause of this is not having a good, clear, big picture of the finished product to reference.

The other day, in training the volleyball team, two big pieces of the puzzle fit into place. We accomplished five times dumbbell complex and fives times half-leg circuit. Now we are ready to add some of the early agility progressions and to move to the next step in the jumping progressions. The reference point is a championship female high school volleyball player.

Perspective

I have attended several meetings where the topic of parents in youth sports came up; in fact it was a recurrent theme. This certainly struck a nerve with me. I think, reflecting back on my 38 years of coaching, one of the biggest things that has changed is the involvement of parents. Thirty-eight years ago a parent would never think to question a coach on anything. Today, the parents are always involved and always questioning. This incessant drive to gain a scholarship or a pro contract has really distorted the whole perspective on youth and high school sports. I certainly was involved as a parent in my daughter's athletic career—sometimes possibly too involved—so I think I can look at this from a personal perspective. Not every kid will get a scholarship; even fewer will play professionally or be Olympians.

Somehow we have to regain a healthy perspective that gives the young athlete space and allows the coaches to do their jobs. On the other hand, it is important for the coaches to be well trained and professional in their approach. We all need to recognize that everyone is not created equal in ability. As the athletes rise through the system, the better athletes will get more playing time and recognition. Everyone cannot be a star, but everyone can strive to be the best they can be.

As adults and coaches we need to stress commitment and individual improvement to the youngsters so they measure against themselves. I realize this is a Pollyanna attitude, but I still believe it. I know who the stars are on the volleyball team I am working with, but as an athletic development coach my greatest satisfaction comes from the young freshman girl who may never play varsity, but has been there every day working extremely hard. In my eyes, she is just as much a star as the stars.

Win the Workout

I first heard this concept, "win the workout," presented by Wayne Goldsmith at the American Swim Coaches convention a few years ago. I immediately found it an intriguing concept and one that has virtually become a mantra for athletes that I work with. Another way to rephrase it, is that it is not so much what you do, but how you do it. The ICE—Intensity, Concentration and Effort—acronym grew out of the concept of winning the workout. ICE gets you in position to win the workout. The essence of it though, is that before you can even think about winning a game, a match or a race, you must win the workout. This is highly individual. I encourage the athletes I work with to ask themselves a simple question after each workout: Did I win the workout? A simple yes or no answer will suffice. This is their responsibility and key to their own personal management. The more workouts you win the better position you put yourself in to win the competition. In pro sports, too often I hear the losers lament that they will turn it on when the lights come on. You can't and won't— you perform the way you practice.

It is a step-by-step process with each training session seamlessly flowing from the training sessions into competition. Here are steps to help with winning the workout:

1. Be clear on what you want to achieve in the workout.

2. Decide on the best methods to help you achieve your goals in the workout.

3. Be sure to measure what you want to achieve.

4. Make sure the workout is in context with the whole plan.

5. Perform the workout with ICE.

6. Evaluate the workout objectively.

Remember, it is a process, a means to an end. Winning the workout is an excellent way to keep your eye on the prize while achieving short-term, incremental progress toward a long-term goal. Go for it!

The System

It's the system, stupid! I have this posted in a prominent place in my office. The system produces results because there is context for all the modes and methods of training. It is more than training muscles and a hodge-podge of exercises. There is a specific sequence and progression that is planned in advance. The athlete's progress is measured against the plan. There is a comfort in this because it is easy to show the athlete if they are on track or behind where they should be at a specific time in the plan.

A system also allows for adjustments that are proactive rather than reactive. All of that being said, the system must have built-in flexibility to adjust to the athlete or the specific situation. If the athlete has to fit into or conform to the system, then there are problems. For example, with the girls' volleyball team I am working with, at the end of the first six-week block we had outstanding jump improvements, but superficially we were not doing much jumping. We actually were, but it was transparent: the foundation strength work we were doing led to the jump improvements. This told me that we were right on schedule and could proceed as planned with the next block. Without the template of the system to compare against, the temptation would be to do more of the same. Remember, it is the system that determines long-term success.

In an issue of the *New York Times* sports magazine, *Play*, there was an interesting article called "How to Build a Prodigy—The Super-Athlete Formula" by Daniel Coyle. It certainly affirmed that success is about the system. The centerpiece of the article was Spartak Tennis Club in Moscow that has produced an inordinate number of top players. I am not a big fan of starting at five-years old, but here is a system that keeps them playing and moves them to the highest level.

Planning

Dwight D. Eisenhower said: "In preparing for battle I have always found that plans are useless, but planning is indispensable." This certainly is applicable to coaching. My experience has taught me that detailed long-term plans are virtually useless; they end up changing so much by the time they are implemented that any resemblance to the original plan is coincidental. That does not mean there is no planning—far from it— but the key is the focus of the plan. I have shifted my focus away from detailed long-term planning to more general thematic plans for the long term and very detailed plans for sessions and microcycles.

Achievement Zones

Not long ago, Steve Odgers, a former athlete, and colleague of mine with the White Sox, visited me at

home. Steve now works for Scott Boras, the most powerful agent in baseball. He does the conditioning for Boras' clients. In that capacity he works with some of the biggest names and highest paid players in baseball. During the visit, Steve and I talked about work, training, achievement, and success. Here are my thoughts based on our conversations: Anyone can work. Work is not training. Training has a specific direction and purpose in pursuit of a specific goal. There are three training zones:

> **Zone One** is the foundation. This is where the athlete starts. They get familiar with training. They learn routine. The work is more general in nature. In essence, they get in a comfort zone.

> **Zone Two** is the performance zone. Here they learn to be uncomfortable. The intensity is higher. There is a narrower focus.

> **Zone Three** is the high-performance zone. This is the zone where many are called and few are chosen. This demands the highest level of commitment. Everything here is purposeful, mindful and directed. There is no fluff. This is where the big dogs play.

Progression from zone to zone is not automatic. There is no social promotion. Each step must be earned. It seems that the hardest transition is getting out of zone one. There are many million-dollar athletes in zone one. They are simply getting by on ability and skill. The great ones—the ones who achieve consistently at the highest levels—live, work and play in zone three.

Vibration Training

Vibration training is the latest fad. The fact that it is a fad bothers me. It is a viable training tool and modality in the correct hands and in the correct situation. It is not viable for the general public in a health club or gym environment without strict supervision. As a method it has been around for at least 30 years. I first saw it alluded to in Soviet training literature in the 1970s.

I did an extensive literature search of vibration training about six years ago and found an article in an *American Physical Therapy* journal from the early '70s. A lot of the early research on vibration was designed to study the negative effects in industrial settings and with truck drivers. Don't quote me on this, but I also think this was a factor that was studied early in the space program due to the severe vibration forces at lift-off. I have not had any first-hand experience using vibration with athletes. I have played with it a bit myself just to get a feel for it.

My colleagues, who have used it in a systematic manner with elite athletes, believe that vibration definitely helps with flexibility. They also feel that it is very individual in its application and adaptive response. Some have used it very individually as a recovery modality. The vibration platforms they used were not commercial platforms, but specially built platforms that had narrower ranges of vibration. I have seen the commercial machines go up in 10 Hz jumps, which is way too big a jump in my opinion. There is also the danger of harmonic convergence with human tissue. If not used properly it can explode eyeballs!

A good overview of vibration training from a scientific perspective is, "Vibration Loads: Potential for Strength and Power Development" by Mester, Spitzenpfeil and Yue, in *Strength And Power In Sport, Second Edition*, edited by Pavo Komi. My advice is, let the buyer beware.

Neutral Spine

Is this another concept that has taken on a life of its own, totally out of context? This seems to be the current buzz with gyms passing out t-shirts that read: Is your spine neutral today? Let's take a step back and look at this in the context of the three movement constants: the body, gravity, and the ground. In the body are we once again taking a subcortical action, the neutral spine position, and making it conscious. This happens as needed; it is not something we can consciously make happen. If we could, then ultimately it would not be beneficial because in movement we must react, not think.

Regarding gravity, we are told to learn the neutral spine position. We must start in a supine position so we can feel the proper alignment of the pelvis to achieve this elusive position. When we are in a supine position are we taking gravity out of the equation? In regard to the ground we are bipedal terrestrial beings who move over the ground off of one foot and onto the other foot. Can we maintain a neutral spine during gait without stiff robotic actions? Once again I feel like a voice crying out in the dark. I do not want to be contrary, but to urge people to use good common sense. The neutral spine is not a position. It is a moment in time, part of a bigger picture.

This post was prompted by a question at my seminar in Seattle. I was demonstrating a squat and at the break someone asked me if I tell the person squatting to keep their spine neutral. As I am sure you would expect, my answer was that I tell them to squat. For some reason this question and several others made me think. I was concerned that my answer had sounded flippant, but that was not the intention.

It made me think of some other questions people have asked about movements that seemed to focus on small or extraneous motions that really did not impact the desired outcome. It dawned on me that someone somewhere was teaching people to be aware of all this stuff. I know the term "stuff" is not too scientific, but stuff does get in the way. Focusing on stuff that is extraneous is robotic. If we were building a robot and we had to program each action, then it would be a whole different story. The body is not a robot; we do run motor programs—some are faulty and some are finely tuned. The body has to constantly solve movement problems presented to it by the environment. Most of the time it finds successful solutions, but sometimes it does not. In either case, it moves on. Movement is flowing and natural, and many of the problems we have today are due to lack of movement. It just seems that having to teach someone neutral spine by putting them in a supine position on the floor or plinth, creates a fundamental disconnect. There is too much of a gap between the supine position and weight bearing on one leg—this is true both for the athlete and for the 82-year old lady next door.

Unfamiliar and unnatural positions will not help the body to solve more complex movement problems. Gravity and the ground treat everyone the same, and gravity always wins! There is a simple solution to all of this—get people moving by bending, reaching, pulling, extending, walking or stepping in short, natural movements that work through all three planes of motion. Good motion occurs through the center of the body. The center is a relay site that smoothes out movement and helps with efficiency. By thinking about the pieces and components, the movement will be robotic, and that is not what we want.

How Much is Too much?

Some coaches, even successful ones, focus on getting their athletes to 100 miles a week. I just do not think that is necessary at the high school level when athletes are growing and developing. That is too much, too soon. It reminds me of the old saying, how do you keep them down on the farm after they have seen Paris? Where do they go from there? How do they progress?

I would rather see a broader foundation of work capacity and athleticism. I know the young Kenyans run a lot of miles, but we must also consider their overall lifestyle. Their success has a lot to do with upward mobility. Our kids today generally do not come from as good a movement base as they did in the past. I say this not to be critical, but to get people to think that there are other approaches. A hundred miles a week is not a magic solution. I have coached high school athletes who certainly were capable of running 100-mile weeks, but I am not sure if they would have been faster. In the mid-'70s there were a large number of athletes who were running 100-plus miles a week, but to my knowledge only one or two eventually achieved world class status. In the 1975 California high school state championship meet, my athlete ran 8:56 in the two-mile run for fifth place. He ran 50 to 55 miles a week. The top four in the meet ranged from 95 to 120 miles a week. Maybe, had he reached that level, he would have run much faster, but I really do not think so. Remember, volume is not a biomotor quality. That being said, I also understand there are many roads to Rome, so choose the one that works for your athletes.

Combine Training

The NFL Combine is the event that, along with Groundhog Day, signifies the arrival of spring. Combine training has become a parlor industry with every ex-player who ever strapped on a helmet and lifted a weight advertising combine training. One article I read about a combine preparation factory in New Jersey stated that they had improved a player's time from 5.4 to 5.1 seconds. Wow! That was really impressive. Why didn't he save his money and stay at his university and work with his track coach? When you run that slowly, anything you do will make you faster.

Since the event is usually televised live on the NFL Network, I propose that the NFL charge naming rights and turn it into a team scoring competition. Each player would wear the colors and logo(s) displayed prominently of the combine preparation group that he worked with. It could be like NASCAR with each preparation group matched up against the others. Score it like a track meet with five or six places per position. Give bonus points for anyone who sets a combine record. Oh, by the way, no points if the athlete does not improve over their times before the combine. No hand times, only electronic times. If there is a tie, then the performance directors would have to race in the 40 to determine a winner. I would get the NFL Network to watch that!

Effort-Based Training

A reader asked me to write about the descriptors we use for teaching percentages of maximum effort for use with interval training. For example, what does 80 percent (or 50, 60, 70, 90 percent) of maximum effort feel like? This question was addressed in Athletic Development. Zach, let me briefly explain the genesis of using verbal descriptors rather than actual percentages for the particular distance. Verbal descriptors are nothing more than indicators of perceived exertion that have been validated by Gunnar Borg, a Swedish researcher.

It seemed to make sense, especially when I was working with team sport athletes who had no sense of pace, even if I would have given them an exact number. They should know what 100 percent is—I tell them it is all-out. How hard would all-out effort be for 30 seconds? Then I ask them to run what they think is 80 percent of that with the understanding that they have to run 12, 16 or 18 repetitions with a 30-second walk. Then I coach it. I do not just hold a stopwatch and blow a whistle. I closely observe how they handle it. Probably in the first few sessions they will undershoot and run more within themselves than you would like. As they get into the swing of things, they come to understand the gradations of effort. Basically 70 percent is a pretty conversational pace if the work-to-rest ratio is 1:1. That is a good starting point.

It is good to have descriptors for the various percentages of effort. The famous Hungarian distance coach Mihay Igloi used that system very effectively. I have borrowed that idea and changed the descriptors based on the population. Generally the descriptors go something like this:

> Easy—60 percent
> Medium Easy—65 to 70 percent
> Medium—75 percent
> Medium Hard—80 percent
> Hard—85 to 90 percent
> Competition or Game Effort—95 to 100 percent

Tournament Play

Another reader of my blog wrote to me about my post on tournament play. He said:

> My principal sport is ultimate Frisbee. The sport is played entirely in a tournament format where it is common to play four to five 90-minute games on Saturday and then one to four games on Sunday. The conditioning needs for an individual game (very high intensity, short duration sprinting and jumping) are at odds with the endurance requirements of tournament play.

For an athlete to be successful they need to be able to perform on the last game of Sunday (finals). Obviously, having a bigger team can help. Do you have thoughts on general ways you'd modify conditioning for adult athletes if all competition took place in the context of tournaments?

John, the good news is that you do not have to compete week after week in an extended competitive season. My advice in preparation for this format is to set up training in revolving three-week cycles. The first cycle would have a speed and power emphasis. The second cycle would have a speed endurance emphasis, and the third cycle would have an aerobic emphasis. Repeat this pattern for nine weeks total leading into the tournament.

The last three weeks (10th, 11th and12th weeks) into the tournament should be more specific with week one of that cycle emphasizing skill and game simulation. Week two should be the highest intensity week of the whole cycle, and week three should taper down and rest up for the tournament.

In the last week be sure to do a good warm-up the day before the tournament. Take Thursday off completely and make Wednesday very light. Tuesday of that week should be a speed endurance day, with Monday a short, sharp aerobic day.

Strength Training For Endurance Sports

The first consideration when looking at endurance sports is the type of strength that is necessary to improve performance. This strength is focused on improving skills involved in the events and efficiency. For example, the goal is to improve an athlete's ability to streamline in the water, or to maintain an aerodynamic position in the saddle producing maximum power per pedal stroke on the bike. The goal may also be the ability to use the ground in running as well as tolerate the amount of running necessary by avoiding impact injuries such as tendonitis.

These demands create a little different approach to strength training than in non-endurance sports. The strength goal is to work on exercise movements that improve posture and alignment, rather than produce force. In swimming, the term, *grip it and rip it* leads to a great deal of inefficiencies in the water.

The goal should be to strengthen the core and the legs, and properly strengthen the upper body so that the athletes can improve their distance per stroke. In cycling, a large part of efficiency is to hold the aero position, which demands a large amount of core strength, stability in the shoulders and obviously functional leg strength. In running, efficiency is a matter of balancing stride length with stride frequency and, depending on the length of the run, requires a huge amount of strength endurance.

As endurance sports have become popular there seems to be a distinct misunderstanding of the role of strength training. Strength training is an umbrella term which includes weight training as one component. There is a mistaken notion that one has to go to the gym to strength train. Over the years, I've evolved the concept of a *weight room without walls* for endurance sports. The no-wall weight room is equipped with sets of dumbbells of 10 to 25 percent of body weight, a sturdy box 12 to 14 inches high, a medicine ball about 3 kg, and a stretch cord. With these items, one can do anything needed to strengthen for improved endurance performance.

Since most endurance athletes participate in their sport on a part-time basis, time is of the essence. The program consists of 20 minutes of strength training three times a week, and ten minutes twice a week with extensive static stretching postexercise. This program should also be part of in-season training and, to obtain optimum results, needs to be done for a minimum of 12 weeks. The method requires a consistent application of a few exercises done with intensity. In my opinion, this program is more important for female athletes because of their hormonal profile and a lesser amount of muscle mass, as opposed to their male counterparts.

The strength-training menu is divided into three different categories: *(1) total body*, which includes pulling/pushing movements and their variations done

with dumbbells (i.e., dumbbell high pull, rotational snatch with
(2) lower extremities, which are all derived from squatting mov
and lunges all done single leg or alternating legs; and *(3) upper body*, which
includes more body weight type of movements such as pull-ups, push-ups and
their variations, and core strength work.

When to Stretch

**There are a lot of experts who now advocate dynamic
stretching and movement as part of warm-up.** Some say that
static stretching even reduces power. In warm-up, the latest research
indicates that static stretching is counterproductive. It has a relaxing effect
but no positive impact on exciting the central nervous system to get the
body ready for training. However, after a workout the calming effect of static
stretching is desirable to get the muscles back to resting state. This is the
logic for static stretching. The recommended time for holding the stretch is
15 to 30 seconds. What I've found is that this type of stretching doesn't have
to be done immediately postexercise. There seems to be a window of about
two to three hours after training to gain the effect you want. I've found that
after a late afternoon workout, one should do a cool down, eat and then
do extensive static stretching. This aids reduction, or at least minimizes the
onset of muscle soreness.

Valery Borzov

**Valery Borzov was the Olympic champion at the 100 and
200 meters.** We will never know what would have happened if the whole
American contingent had made it to the starting line for the 100 meters
in Munich. Borzov certainly was on top of his game at the Olympics and
he clearly beat the best in the 200 meters. I got to see Borzov run once
indoors and at the '76 Olympics where he took the bronze in the 100 meters.
Technically, he was impressive. That was the first time a sprinter had medaled
in the 100 meters in two Olympics.

Much mythology has arisen around Borzov. He is one of the few male sprinters to come out of the Soviet Union; they had success with females, but not the same success with the males. At age 15, a comparable age to an American high school sophomore or junior, he ran a 10.7 hundred meters. That certainly shows very good potential. He was very well coached by Valetin Petrovsky. He did not run that many meets so he was able to point for the big meets, where he usually excelled.

In contrast to other Soviet sprinters before him, he did not look like a weight lifter. I used to marvel at the Soviet sprinters in the '60s who looked more like weight lifters than sprinters. They were always great for 30 or 40 meters and then would fade. It is only speculation, but perhaps he was identified young and trained properly as a sprinter, with a proper balance instead of an emphasis on maximum strength. What I have read of his coach makes a lot of sense—he was very forward thinking then and quite contemporary today. Mind you, this is all my opinion because there continues to be a veil of mystery surrounding Borzov. To my knowledge, no Western writer has interviewed him. It would be enlightening to see someone do that and find out details of his training and background.

Swimming for Baseball Conditioning

Another reader of my blog wrote to ask me my thoughts on swimming in shorter bursts as a form of conditioning for pitchers. There are certainly much better alternatives.

Pitching is a ballistic, dynamic activity. Swimming is not. In addition, the pitcher would have to be a pretty good swimmer to get enough out of the swimming, and the additional stress on the shoulder is not worth the risk. Power activities and intensity are the stimulus for improving and conditioning pitchers. Some water running would be good for recovery as well as some upper-body, large amplitude movements in chest-deep water.

One thing to watch in the water is the effect that it has on the callus buildup on a pitcher's fingers. The water may soften the callus, which could affect the movement of the ball. Another thought is that if the pitcher lives near the ocean, surfing is great. The paddling is a great motion and the balance required is fantastic, although there is still a bit of concern on the callus issue. To substitute for surfing, I have always used the Vasa Swim Trainer with my pitchers. I noticed way back when I first started coaching, that the kids who were the surfers excelled in the softball throw, which was part of the President's Physical Fitness Test then. I was talking to Rob Sleamaker about it. He is the inventor of the Vasa (http://www.vasatrainer.com), so he sent me a Vasa to use with the White Sox. The pitchers loved it. I put it into the program and varied the routine based on the time of the season. We got the advantages of surfing without the water. I actually use it in many of my strength-training programs.

Teaching and Coaching

Coaching and teaching are essentially the same—sharing and raising the standard of performance along with the level of expectation. They are also about finding the correct buttons to push, given varied styles of learning, innate ability and motivation. Not every athlete engages in a sport to be an athlete. Often, the younger athletes do not even know what that is. Our job as coaches is to teach good training habits along with sound fundamentals. Some will want to achieve at higher levels and others will not. The trick is to serve both without short changing either. Many young boys and girls just want the affiliation of being part of a team, and we must not forget that. Some of my fondest coaching memories are of these athletes.

Athleticism

Where have all the athletes gone? At first that may seem like a very naïve statement, but let's examine it further. Look beyond the numbers, and the spectacular performances at the elite levels of sport. What is missing? It is athleticism. We know it when we see it. We talk about it, but do we know how to develop it? What is it?

Let's begin by defining the term. Given its widespread use I was surprised that I was unable to find an acceptable definition, so I came up with the following definition of athleticism. Athleticism is the ability to execute athletic movements at optimum speed with precision, style and grace. It is certainly not a very complicated definition. It is easy to see when someone has it. It is certainly inherent in successful performers in any sport. My observation is that in sport, even though performance standards continue to skyrocket, we are seeing less and less athleticism, especially at the developmental levels. With increased early specialization and an emphasis on specificity we have sacrificed overall athleticism.

Rethinking Core Training

The fundamental underlying philosophy is that all training is core training. Without a fully functioning core, efficient movement is not possible. The core is involved in all movement as a major factor in the control of movement. Currently core training is the buzzword in training. We need to rethink how we are training the core in the light of the above-stated philosophy. Conventional wisdom would have us doing much of our training in prone and supine positions while emphasizing drawing in or sucking in of the stomach muscles in order to activate the internal oblique and transverse abdominis. That is fine in theory, but in practice we need to look at how the core functions as one of the largest links in the kinetic chain.

The body is a link system. This link system is referred to as the kinetic chain. Functional core training is all about taking advantage of this linkage. It is how all the parts of the chain work together in harmony to produce smooth, efficient patterns of movement. Movement occurs from toenails to fingernails with all the segments working in harmony to produce smooth, efficient movement.

In order to truly understand core function in the context of whole-body function, we must shift our focus away from individual muscles to integrated movements. Current thinking would have us focus on the transverse abdominis and the internal oblique as key core muscles. This is fallacious thinking because the brain does not recognize individual muscles. Those muscles are two core muscles among many that contribute to efficient core function.

The brain recognizes patterns of movement, which consist of the individual muscles working in harmony to produce movement. It is unreasonable to think that two muscles could play such an important role that they are more important than any other muscle. According to Stuart McGill in his book *Low Back Disorders—Evidence-Based Prevention and Rehabilitation*, pg. 144:

> The muscular and motor control system must satisfy requirements to sustain postures, create movements, brace against sudden motion or unexpected forces, build pressure and assist challenged breathing, all while ensuring sufficient stability. Virtually all muscles play a role in ensuring stability, but their importance at any point in time is determined by the unique combination of the demands just listed.

Shin Splints and Compartment Surgery

A reader wrote to ask me this:

> I would like to get your thoughts on something. I just got off the phone with a girl who has been playing field hockey at Princeton and her career is being threatened by lower compartment syndrome. She had the release surgery and it did not help much, as of yet. She has a friend who plays D1 soccer who has the same thing. She told me also that she ran into a D1 field hockey coach at another major university who said this is becoming epidemic (shin splints, lower compartment, etc.). What are your thoughts on this?

This surgery was quite the rage a few years ago. I actually thought it had gone out of favor. This is a classic example of reductionist medicine—focusing on the symptom rather than taking a giant step back and looking at the big picture. Because there is pain and swelling there, you operate. Bottom line is that nine times out of ten, the operation does not work. Think globally— look above and below the problem. I am of the opinion that the problem really stems from the inability to properly shock absorb. The big shock absorber that needs to be developed is the buttocks. Movement mechanics must be addressed, such as how they stop and change direction. Look at the foot—more specifically, is the subtalar joint locked up?

As far as the shin splint issue, it is much the same answer. I know field hockey must play on a very firm and generally unforgiving surface, so look at opportunities to train off the surface for non-technical work. Look at footwear. I have found that rigid shoes are often the culprit. In collegiate and national team environments, the players are often forced to wear a sponsor's shoes and all of one style. That shoe and style may not be correct for the individual athlete. The common solution for shin splints is to do dorsiflexion exercises, which can cause more harm than good because the anterior tibialis' main job is to help decelerate the foot. Once again, work above and below.

Excessive weight is another issue, but it's tough to address with the female athlete. When they are too heavy, gravity wins. Not an easy problem to solve, but with work it can be done.

Train for Work Capacity Not Endurance

We have all heard the axiom that more is not necessarily better. But within each of us there is a fundamental insecurity that we are not doing enough, so we do extra work. This seems to be especially true in an endurance-dominated event. The result is that we lose sight of our objective in training, which is to become a faster cyclist, runner or swimmer. The work should not be an end in itself but a means to an end. That end is the improvement of performance. All training should be in pursuit of this objective.

Work capacity is the ability to tolerate a high workload and to recover sufficiently for the next workout or competition. Raising work capacity will improve the athlete's capacity to resist fatigue. It involves the functional efficiency and coordination of the cardiovascular, metabolic and nervous systems. With all these systems working together, work capacity is closely related to speed, strength, flexibility and coordination. It is more than endurance. An increase in work capacity will allow the athlete to work more efficiently and get more out of each training session. In the language of training theory, it is General Physical Preparation (GPP) type of work.

In order to raise work capacity with the objective of improving performance it is necessary to incorporate a mix of three elements:

1. Capacity—the total amount of energy available to perform work.
2. Power—amount of energy that can be produced per unit of time.
3. Efficiency—optimal use of the energy available.

The tendency is to emphasize capacity to the exclusion of power and efficiency. To be most effective, a blend of all three is best, depending on the individual athlete's strengths and weaknesses, and the particular sport they are preparing for. The most overlooked of the three, and yet the one that has the most potential for improvement, is efficiency. Improving efficiency allows greater utilization of the capacity and power available.

This is achieved through proper periodization, which is essentially having a plan and working with that plan. Also, detailed record-keeping is critical to provide objective feedback. Know yourself by honestly assessing your strengths and weaknesses. Know your sport. Ask yourself how you have achieved the best results.

Conceptually this all seems very simple, and it is, but putting it into practice is tough. It is much easier to fall back into the security of quantification rather than the preparation to compete.

Questions on Training and Fitness

The following are common questions and concerns from coaches on training and fitness:

When is it appropriate to begin formal speed training?

A common mistake many coaches make when beginning formal speed training is to prepare their players for a track meet and not for the game that they are training for. Speed training for sport should always have a game-like emphasis. Typically, younger players between the ages of seven to nine should focus on free play. Variations of games such as tag are a wonderful way to work on speed and improve gross motor skills.

Coaching considerations prior to implementing any type of formal training include the ability of the player to handle formal instruction and the player's physical maturity level. Starting at an early age, sport technique should be developed concurrently with speed training. Once these skills have been mastered, players need to learn to distribute their efforts relative to the technical and tactical demands of the game, incorporating short, explosive bursts with varied changes of direction.

I need to improve my team's endurance. Should I do distance running?

Practical experience and research have shown that slow, steady distance running detracts from speed and explosiveness. In the last minutes of a game or match your players should not only be able to run, but continue to run fast. This is accomplished by incorporating fartleks and interval runs into your training. For example, have your players perform a 30/30 run. This is a 30-second jog followed by a 30-second run at 70 percent of maximal effort. Carefully consider the conditioning that also occurs in the course of practice. Additional fitness work that is relative to the demands of the game and properly planned into the overall training cycle will help to ensure a fitter and faster team.

When is it appropriate to begin formal strength training for a young player?

Strength is one of the biggest deficiencies in young athletes. As with speed training, the athlete's emotional development and level of physical maturity are important in determining if the athlete can learn the routines and handle formal training. Although research has shown that prepubescent athletes may benefit from weight training, heavy loading of the spine is not recommended until after puberty. The player has to be able to handle his or her own body weight before adding external resistance. This can be accomplished by incorporating push-ups, pull-ups, body weight lunges, and body weight squats into your program. Various medicine ball exercises, as well as hopping and jumping games will also help to strengthen the tendons and ligaments further, helping to prevent injury and establishing a solid strength base.

How can I include fitness activities within a normal practice?

Integrate each component throughout the entire practice. It all starts with a proper warm-up. This is the time to work on balance, coordination, speed work and high quality touches on the ball. The objective is to work up to game effort speed, therefore, warm up to play, don't play to warm up.

From this point on, the entire practice should mimic the game. This requires a well-thought-out training plan that flows from one component to the next with a smooth transition. For example, when performing team drills, the length of the lines affects the work-to-rest ratio. Players should never stand around for more than 30 to 40 seconds at a time. Use the length of the lines to determine the desired work-to-rest ratio. We look at the whole practice as a water break. Have your players bring their own water bottle so that whenever they need a break, they quickly take it and get immediately back into practice.

What can I do to help prevent fatigue when my team plays two games in one day?

Your players are only as good as their ability to recover. Factors such as hydration and a pre- and post-nutrition plan are always important. Be aware of environmental conditions such as altitude changes, time zone changes, and the weather. The warm-up before the first game will be more extensive while the warm-up before the second game will be much shorter in duration. Many teams will go through a long warm-up before their second game and end up coming out flat. This may be attributed to the players becoming fatigued from the long, second warm-up. Include a cool down after each game lasting approximately 10 to 15 minutes, incorporating light jogging and dynamic flexibility. End the cool down with a short, static stretching routine to help the muscles return to resting length.

Discipline: An Outdated Concept?

I spend a lot of time with friends who are coaches. Invariably the topic turns to today's athletes, and to one question: "Are they different?"

They certainly are different in many ways from the athletes of 1969, when I started coaching. But the biggest differences are not in the athletes themselves, but in the society we live in.

One of those differences has been a breakdown in discipline. Discipline is the foundation for excellence, and self-discipline is the highest form of discipline.

Of course, for youngsters to learn self-discipline they must have guidance— what is right, and what is not right? That guidance takes the form of rules.

Coaches today have become reluctant to set rules, because then they must enforce them. That could be uncomfortable. What if a parent challenges them? Will they receive backing from the administration, from the school board, the principal, the vice-principal, and the athletic director? That's certainly a legitimate concern, when anything from an attack by a parent, to the coach's job, to a lawsuit could be at stake.

My conversations with various coaches who have been coaching for more than 20 years indicate that such backing from the school system, or lack of it, is the basic problem.

Coaches believe in discipline just as they always have, but they do not have the backing they used to have. Younger coaches are reluctant to set rules and enforce discipline because they will not be popular and they know they will not be backed.

What is the answer? Sport is not isolated from society; it is a microcosm of the society in which we live. So it is naïve to think that the problems that exist in society will not exist on our sport teams.

Learning discipline demands guidance. We, as coaches, must provide that guidance. We must set the standards using fair rules that carefully lay out the behavioral expectations involved in being part of the team. These must be written. They must be clear so that there is no room for debate. Essentially, as the coach, you are providing a structure to begin to improve their abilities and their enjoyment of the sport.

I think many of today's athletes crave the structure we can give them, even though it may not be part of their everyday lives outside of sport. But they have to understand that it's a two-way street—they can't just follow the rules they like. Sometimes they must obey the rules they don't like. That's the price they have to pay for the structure the coach provides.

Discipline is a responsibility of coaching. If we do not enforce discipline then we are shirking our duty as coaches.

We must understand that we are not coaching a sport; we are coaching young men and women who are competing in a sport. We owe it to them to provide the most positive experience that we can. Through firm and fair discipline we can create a favorable learning environment that will allow them to reach their potential.

How can we do this? We can start by getting everyone on our side.

You and your coaching staff should decide on the behavior that you expect of your athletes and then set the rules that will define those behaviors. Review them with your athletic director and if need be, the principal. Get them to buy in and support you before any challenges are made. It might be even better if you can get your athletic department to set rules that members of every team at your school must observe, to ensure consistency from sport to sport. To those general rules, you can add rules specific to your sport. And if you feel comfortable doing so, you might want to involve the senior athletes and the parents in the process. If they're part of the process, it's easier for them to buy in.

Once the rules are set, schedule a mandatory parents meeting to go over the rules and responsibilities for their youngsters to be on the team. This meeting should also help the parents learn about practice procedures, nutrition guidelines, lettering policy and criteria for varsity selection. Take the opportunity to educate the parents about the sport.

Both the parent and the child must sign a statement that they will observe the rules. If they do not, they will not be allowed to participate. Emphasize that to be an athlete is special. It is a privilege to participate, not a right. There should also be a pledge from the coaches as to the behavioral standards the athletes and parents can expect from the coach. The ultimate goal is to create an atmosphere of mutual respect.

Remember, as coaches we have a responsibility to teach our athletes. Very few will compete past the high school level, but they all can have the great growing-up experiences of testing their limits and being part of a team.

Discipline will help ensure a positive experience. It is not outdated, and it never will be.

Crossing the T's and Dotting the I's

As a young coach I was always told to be sure to cross the T's and dot the I's. At first I thought they were kidding me, but the longer I coached the more I realized that there was much truth attached to that time-worn cliché. Here are some T's to cross and I's to dot that I have found to be important in my own coaching, and through observation of successful coaches and athletes during the past 38 years.

Talent—It all begins here. Without native athletic ability and a feel for the event, it is tough for an athlete to excel at the highest levels. That doesn't mean that someone with less talent can't succeed, but he or she will have to work much harder. The less talented individual will also have less margin for error in training. The coach's job is to identify, nurture and direct the talent.

Tenacity—Mental toughness is the result of sound physical preparation. It is also the ability to focus on the task at hand and not be distracted by minor setbacks. The champion is often the one who can persevere and overcome obstacles.

Technique—Sound, fundamental movement skills are a precursor to specific event technique. Both must be developed early in an athlete's career and refined as the athlete progresses to the elite level. The challenge is to become technically proficient without becoming mechanical.

Training—This is the process of acquiring specific fitness while balancing all training components. Obviously, this is the foundation for success. No one can succeed without a good training base. Never lose sight of the fact that training is a means to an end, not an end unto itself. That end is competition. Winning is the outcome of good preparation.

Tactics—Tactics are based on knowledge of the sport and on effective competitive skills. Know the rules; study the skills involved in competing well.

Testing—The competition is the ultimate test of the total training program. It must be measured not only by wins and losses, but also by improvement and quality of effort. In order to be ready for the ultimate test, it is important to test periodically in training to assess progress toward a goal.

Inspiration—This is the spark that motivates the coach and the athlete to persevere through difficult times. It is the vision of the results of the hard work. It is the courage to do the little things that make the best better. It is the willingness to do the morning run when it is snowing and it would be easier to stay in bed. It is doing the cool down after a very hard workout when it would be easier to head for the shower. Inspiration is the guiding light toward pursuit of the goal.

Innovation—The willingness to try new things, to change even if you have been successful. Change is a constant. We must be willing to change to get better. This involves continually learning and upgrading your knowledge base. Never be satisfied with where you are now; always seek ways that will help you get better.

Intensity—This is the laser-like focus on the task at hand, the focus that is necessary to be the best you can be. In coaching it is not screaming and hollering; it is focus, concentration and inner drive. It is attention to detail.

Interest—This is the commitment to improve. Your interest must be clearly defined—it is to be the best coach or athlete you can be. The interest must be unwavering.

Involvement—This is necessary for success in any endeavor. You must be fully involved; it cannot be a passing fancy. Involvement is a twenty-four-hour commitment, not a two-hour commitment during the workout. It is committing to a lifestyle that supports excellence. Everyone wants to be involved on meet day, but the winners are those coaches and athletes who pay the price everyday.

Teaching Movement

The key is letting kids explore the dimensions that their bodies can move in. The prime ages for this are the so-called *skill hungry* years, ages seven to nine. Set up games and situations that elicit the movements that you want to see. For example, match colored dots or shapes on the floor with a particular task needed for each color or shape. Simple cues like, run loud or run quiet, will help them learn different foot strikes through discovery. I always use the analogy of *Karate Kid, Part One*: "Wax on, wax off!"

Creativity

The following was posted on Seth Godin's blog (http://sethgodin.typepad.com):

Ninety-nine percent of the time, in my experience, the hard part about creativity isn't coming up with something no one has ever thought of before. The hard part is actually executing the thing you've thought of.

It made me think that too often we try to be original when what is more important is to stick with what is known and proven and build upon that. I know some of the most creative ideas I have had about training came in the middle of a session when I had to solve a problem with a movement in a particular athlete, or even as simple a thing as having to adapt because I didn't have enough medicine balls. Little things like that have triggered some significant changes and adaptations. It makes me think of a line from one of my favorite Texas Tornado songs, *A Little Bit is Better than Nada*, and sometimes you want the whole enchilada.

Stretching is NOT Warm-up

How clear can that be? Yet, I still see teams wallow around on the ground for ten or fifteen minutes at the start of practice to warmup. We certainly know better, but this is still a prevalent practice. When someone pulls a muscle it is usually blamed on the fact that they did not stretch enough before training. How absurd! I always use the analogy of the cat or dog who wakes up from a nap; they do not stretch, they move slowly and rhythmically first through progressively bigger ranges of motion. If they are scared out of a dead sleep they burst away.

A few years ago, this was the topic in a roundtable and Art Venegas, the track and field coach at UCLA put it quite well, "How many times do you see someone stealing hub caps on a car, pull a muscle? It is pure fight or flight, and all they are thinking about is getting the heck out of there. I kind of doubt they stretched for 20 minutes beforehand."

There is a lesson here. If you are spending more than two to three minutes static stretching as part of your warm-up, you are wasting time. Flexibility work has a definite place in a comprehensive training program. The flexibility work should be based on individual needs, not group stretching.

Fit to Test or Fit to Play?

There is a real and distinct difference on the one hand and some real lessons to be learned on the other. It all depends how the fitness tests are used and how they are framed in the overall context of the annual and career plan. The goal, in a competitive environment, is accurate feedback of the physical qualities that could determine success in the game. Selection and timing of tests sends a message. Therefore, decide what message you want to send. If you are going to use a two- or three-mile run test upon reporting, then you are sending a message to the team that it is an endurance sport and they need to get ready for that. The game could be the opposite, but if their place on the team depends on it they will train for the test!

Teaching Athleticism

There is a saying that, "You don't need to see different things, but rather to see things differently." Sometimes we overlook the obvious. In the incessant search to improve performance we have gotten away from the essence of it all—the foundation of athleticism. It can be developed through a systematic approach to athlete development. It is imperative to look for every opportunity to incorporate elements of athleticism in all aspects of training.

Specific sport skills are a combination of patterns of complex motor programs. They are patterns that can be reproduced when we tap into the wisdom of the body. Through experiencing all different patterns of movement we learn to let things happen. We learn to let the motor program run. We cue an action that will result in a chain reaction of efficient movement. We need to emphasize a free play approach that results in fluidity and improvisational skills.

Should we try to teach every movement and then coach it? Or should we allow the athlete the joy of discovery through exploration? There seems to be a worry about them getting it wrong. My answer to that is, what is wrong? There must be spontaneity, a joy and anticipation in movement, a sense of discovery of sport skills and training, not a robotic programmed approach.

It has been my experience working with athletes at all levels, in a wide variety of sports, that athletes will find their own best way of doing something if they are put in a position where they have to adapt. Each athlete has a *movement signature*. It is their stamp, their personal interpretation of the skill. They are very adaptable. We need to encourage an extemporaneous approach, much like great jazz improvisation.

What has caused this? There are several factors:

1. Early specialization in one event is a serious problem that has contributed to the decline of athleticism. The broader range of motor skills developed through free play and exposure to many varied motor programs is a big limiting factor. The choice is to produce better all-around athletes or produce highly concentrated one-sport specialists with very narrow skill ranges. Ultimately, the goal is to produce the best athlete possible with a rich repertoire of motor skills to select from, to better execute the specific sport skill.

2. One-sided training with an emphasis on one or two components of performance rather than a blend. The components of performance, and therefore training, are: speed, strength, stamina, suppleness, skill and recovery. There is a synergistic relationship between all components;

therefore, all components must be trained during all phases of the year in varying combinations.

3. Monkey-see, monkey-do syndrome. Just because an athlete has been successful with a particular training method does not mean the method is the best or should be copied. It is my experience that many athletes are successful in spite of, not because of, their training. Make sure that what you are doing is based on sound training principles and a good progression. Above all, make sure it fits the athletes you are presently working with.

4. Nobody gets hurt, but nobody gets better. Training that is so conservative or narrow that the athlete is never challenged, will not produce results. This is the justification for many machine-oriented strength training programs. Some feel that they are safe when in fact, because they fail to challenge the athleticism of the athlete, they might actually predispose the athlete to injury.

It is always easy and convenient to look to the *good old days* as being better. The simple fact is, that before the advent of specialization, athletes learned and competed in several sports. It was not unusual to see a high school athlete compete in three or four sports. This was not so bad. The athlete may not have been as good early on, but once they did choose to specialize they had a broader base of motor skills to draw upon to enhance their chosen sport skill. Sometimes it is good to look back in order to gain perspective and move ahead. We cannot go backward, but we must look for ways to enhance athleticism that has been lost due to early specialization.

Assessing Force Reduction

Initially, I use a lunge test. Look at the difference in distance right to left, and look at the ability to smoothly return to starting position without deviations. You can also look at the lateral lunge for frontal plane and then rotational lunge for transverse plane. I also use a hop and stick test. Hop for distance and stick the landing and hold for five seconds; repeat with the other leg. They should be able to absorb ankle/knee/hip.

Two-Foot or One-Foot Jump?

Why do some people prefer to jump off of two feet and others off of one? Back in the mid-1980's, when I was working with the Bulls, I saw it up close. Charles Oakley could not jump off of one foot. Tex Winter, one of the assistants, felt it was really hindering him. We tried a bunch of ideas to try to get him to jump off of one foot, but under pressure he always reverted. Conversely, in testing vertical jump on the Vertec with Michael Jordan, he was terrible off of two feet. When he took a step and went off of one foot the difference was unbelievable. In short, I think it represents a personal preference and may represent where you play on the floor. Certainly with young kids I think it advisable to devise games that encourage all types of take-offs.

Play on One Leg or Train on One Leg?

I am an advocate of single-leg squats and unilateral and reciprocal training exercises of the lower extremity (and for that matter, the upper body also). When you consider the forces that players must attenuate on one leg in stopping and starting it makes sense to train unilaterally.

Also, consider the phenomenon of bilateral transfer in doing work with one limb. Bilateral transfer refers to the phenomenon of improvement in function of one limb by working on the opposite limb. This is based on the contralateral function of the brain hemispheres in controlling movement through both cortical and subcortical impulses, that enable movement to be transferred from one side of the body to the other side. That does not mean that squats are not part of the routine—they are, but when and where in the program is the key. Single leg squats, lunges and step-ups and step-downs are the constants because essentially, in most sports, the movement is off of one leg and onto the other leg in multiple directions and in multiple planes.

The strength work must be closely coupled with multi-dimensional speed and agility work to add the speed element to the high force element. This also has an implication for testing. We need to test strength on one leg, stability on one leg, and the ability to reduce force on one leg. If an athlete is deficient then they must be given remedial work to correct the deficiency, and their actual training drills and exercises must be modified. If not, the risk of injury rises significantly as well as ingraining incorrect movement patterns.

Conditioning Considerations for Tournament Play

I think it is important to state my bias up-front. I am not in favor of tournament play at any level except for the state, regional or national championship play. Tournaments have no place at the younger developmental ages. Here are my reasons:

> 1. Cumulative fatigue severely compromises technical elements and quality of play.

> 2. Cumulative fatigue predisposes the player to injury both in contact and non-contact situations.

> 3. Tournaments compromise the player's overall development because it can take up to a week for a player to fully recover, therefore a vital week of training is lost.

The ideal is for the player to play one game a week, which represents the ideal ratio of training to game play of four to five training days for every game day. Unfortunately, this is not the case, so I will give some practical pointers to help you better prepare your players for tournament play from a conditioning perspective. To get optimum return from your team's participation I suggest you enter into the tournament with one of the following specific objectives:

- To develop the players for championship play by simulating the environment of a playoff situation.
- To expose or "showcase" players.
- To win.

Having these specific objectives as part of a season plan will allow you to evaluate the performance in the context of the whole season.

Obviously, the conditioning goal throughout the year is to prepare the player to play the entire match or game at the highest degree of efficiency with the least amount of fatigue. Tournament play should not compromise that goal. Therefore, actual conditioning should not be altered in specific preparation for tournament play.

A vital point is to remember that you are not conditioning so much for actual play as you are for the ability to recover adequately between games, in order to play effectively in the next game. The specific conditioning considerations are more of a management issue during the actual tournament. The significant training implications are the reduction in the quality of training in the week(s) following the tournament. The following are the intra-tournament considerations that can make an appreciable difference for your player in the course of the tournament:

1. **Warm-up**—The warm-up before the first game of the day should be the longest and most complete. Each subsequent warm-up does not have to be as extensive unless there are more than five hours between games.

2. **Cool down**—This is a must. It should incorporate movement through large ranges of motion as well as static stretching.

3. **Pre-event nutrition**—Be sure to eat. In many tournament situations that I have seen, with early morning games the players try to sleep longer and do not rise early enough to eat. They begin the tournament in a depleted state that only gets worse as the tournament progresses. What each player eats is very individual.

4. **Intra-event nutrition**—In the second and possibly third game of the day, one quarter of a sports bar; at half or during a substitution, with water, can help keep energy levels up.

5. **Post-event nutrition**—Get carbohydrates into the system within the first 20 to 30 minutes after the game. Research has shown that taking advantage of this window can significantly help maintain glycogen stores.

6. **Hydration**—Drink as much as possible starting the night before. During any break in the action, drink. Water is okay. If you use a sports drink carefully look at the sugar content.

7. **Between-game recovery/regeneration**—Above all, get off your feet; if there is adequate time between games, five to ten minutes in a swimming pool can really help.

8. **Between-day recovery/regeneration**—Use a whirlpool followed by a dip in a swimming pool as close after the last game of the day as possible. Be sure to eat foods high in carbohydrates.

Know your players:
- What are their fitness levels?
- How physically mature are they?
- How well do they recover?
- What is their skill level?

Carefully monitor minutes played. Use the tournament as a learning tool to gain information about your players and your team. What is each player's response to fatigue as the tournament progresses? Who gets stronger? Whose performance drops off due to fatigue? This is a plus in that it can give quick, directed feedback, enabling you to adjust your plan for the remainder of the season.

2010 Soccer Odyssey

The opportunity to work with several MLS teams and the U.S. World Cup team from January through May of 1998 gave me a good opportunity to closely observe soccer at the highest levels in this country. In addition, I worked extensively with the physical preparation of youth teams and individuals. I am not claiming that these experiences make me an expert but they gave me a perspective to evaluate soccer in this country, from the developmental level to the professional level. The ideas I present here are based on my experiences with other sports and what I have personally seen in soccer.

If we truly wish to compete with the rest of the world we must seek to identify and develop the best soccer athletes. Yet a six-month study commissioned to examine the sport in 1998 completely ignored this vital area and it continues to be ignored today. There is a big distinction between identifying and training the best soccer players. How many times during the World Cup did I hear the lament that what we need are some Michael Jordans to play soccer. The implication is that we do not get the best athletes to play soccer. We may not have the absolute best, but what we get is pretty good. However, we don't emphasize the development of the physical qualities that support (underlie) the skill. We must find and train fast explosive players who have skill. The physical qualities that underlie soccer skills can be significantly improved, but they must also be trained.

I have had the opportunity for 38 years to prepare teams and individuals for the highest levels of competition in amateur and professional sport. The key to success at any level is a five-component process:

1. The sport and positions.
2. The individual player.
3. The plan.
4. The system.
5. The evaluation.

It is a simple paradigm, and if you study successful teams and nations, all those elements are evident. Just to compete in 2010 and beyond, much less win, we must train the complete soccer athlete.

Soccer is acknowledged as a skill-dominant sport, but several key statistics from match analysis should force us to take another look at time with the ball, and frequency of intensity of effort. This should lead us to question how we train. Are we preparing for the game as it is played in this country or are we preparing for the game as it is played at the World Cup level? The facts are irrefutable, but we must face facts and prepare for the game as it is being played at the world level.

The theme is, train to play. The converse to this is the current approach of playing to train. The prevalent attitude is that more games and more tournaments make the players better. We need to modify this approach. That has gotten us to this point, but if we want to get better, then we have to use this as a starting point and move on. Change is not always comfortable, but it is a constant in life. Let's make change for the better.

We need to develop and refine the concept of the soccer conditioning specialist. The roles and responsibilities of a support person are:

- Planning.
- Recovery and regeneration.
- Speed.
- Strength/power.
- Fitness.
- Liaison with sports medicine staff.

There should be a support person with every national team implementing a consistent program designed to work on athleticism.
Soccer is a high-speed game of skill. It presents a myriad of physical demands, some of which are seemingly contradictory. The first is that if we get good athletes to play we would be better. My contention is that we get

athletes to play, but we ignore their athleticism and train them to be soccer players, not soccer athletes. Athleticism must be developed, sharpened and refined in parallel with soccer skill, tactics and strategy. The most precious quality that a soccer player can possess is speed. Most soccer training programs do not put an emphasis on this component or if they do, it is track speed drills, which do not transfer to the starting, stopping, multi-directional demands of the game.

The second demand is counteracting the monkey-see, monkey-do syndrome. After watching the World Cup, I was even more infatuated with the Dutch style of play and their training methods. But is the solution to improving soccer performance copying the Dutch system, or any other successful system for that matter? In women's collegiate soccer everyone is trying to emulate the UNC program, but that is a program that works at UNC with the coaches, players and system that was refined for that environment.

The lesson is that we must develop our own program based on the step-to-success model. We have a larger population, geographic size, cultural and regional diversity than Holland. Those should be strengths, not weaknesses. What works in Holland, a small country with a sophisticated coaching education program, will not work the same way here. That does not mean, however, that we cannot take elements of their system and incorporate them into ours.

There is already a comprehensive licensing system available. It appears to be an effective system in terms of technical, tactical and strategic preparation, but what about physical preparation, periodization and long-term planning? This is where our system breaks down. We need to do a better job of preparing our coaches or, at the very least, develop a sub-specialization within the existing process that prepares the coach in all aspects of physical preparation, planning, and recovery and regeneration. We need to do this to catch up to the rest of the world.

Coaching Talent Search

I am starting a coaching talent search. It has been disappointing to witness a trend in the placement of athletic development coaches who lack the proper coaching skills and possess scant expertise. Since I quite often receive requests asking for recommendations for jobs, I have decided to address this by starting a clearinghouse for those athletic development professionals who fit the profile outlined below. This *will not be* a placement service, and there will be no fee for this. My goal here is to help define the profession and help good, qualified people attain placement in positions where they can use their knowledge and advance the profession. Do not send anything if you do not meet the profile. Please do not call me. If there is a job opportunity I will have the prospective employer contact you. I am looking for remarkable people who will make an impact in this field.

Athletic Development Coach Profile

Statement of philosophy of training and coaching (two paragraphs maximum).

Specific short-term and long-term goals.

Education and relevant course work.

All coaching experience, in any sport at any level.
    Specifically, who did you coach?
    What were your responsibilities?

Teaching experience—formal and informal.

Areas of coaching expertise—be specific.

What are your strengths? What makes you special and stand out from your peers?

What are your weaknesses? Where do you need to improve? How do you plan to address your weaknesses?

Appearance—Do you look the part? Are you fit and do you present yourself well?

Skill proficiency—Do you have the ability to demonstrate what you are teaching?

Work ethic—Are you willing to go the extra mile and work until the job is done?

Certifications and accreditations—List all in any field.

List three books on training or athletic enhancement that you have read in the past three months.

List three journal articles that you have read in the last three months.

What are you doing on a regular basis to improve your knowledge and ability as a coach?

Specialization

In a recent issue of *Atlantic Magazine*, Robert Kaplan wrote an article titled, "Thucydides: A Historian for Our Time" about the historian Herodotus. Kaplan is the Distinguished Visiting Professor in National Security at the United States Naval Academy and a regular contributor to *Atlantic*. The quote below jumped out at me as particularly relevant. This pinpoints a major problem that we have today in medicine, athletic development, athletic training and, for that matter, in everyday life.

In the Academy (Naval Academy), specialization has become both a necessity and a curse. Too much narrow expertise is the inverse of wisdom. But the explosion of facts that need to be categorized demands a growing number of parochial subdivisions within any given field. We must fight against the tendency to become, as the Spanish philosopher José Ortega y Gasset feared we all would, 'learned ignoramuses.'

Today, I see more people specializing in narrower and narrower areas. I am so thankful for the guidance that I received early in my coaching career that steered me toward being a generalist. When I wanted to become a track coach, Red Estes, then the assistant track coach at Fresno State suggested that I train for the decathlon, that way I would learn all the events. I would experience it first hand. That was the best advice I received. It allowed me to make connections, and to question some of the conventional wisdom in each individual event. I quickly found out what worked and did not work. I learned how to be efficient in my use of training time. I learned the importance of intensity.

Today, it seems everyone wants to be a distance coach. I watch the distance coaches at the USAT&F (USA Track and Field) Level III schools and they act like the other events have the plague. This is a great example of an event group that needs to go to the jumps and sprints to understand the broader dimensions of training. The same can be said about many areas; too many strength coaches only know strength. I am shocked to find out how many strength coaches have *never* gone to talk to the track coaches at their schools. Get out—see and experience the world. Do not be afraid to explore what you don't know. Know what you know and do not know. Get off the Internet and read; read journals in all fields, not just athletic development. It is amazing what you will learn.

A Great Coaching Book

***How Breakthroughs Happen: The Surprising Truth About How Companies Innovate* by Andrew Hargadon.** This is a must-read for all coaches. I know you think I have finally lost it, because the title doesn't say anything about coaching. That is precisely why it is a good coaching book. As coaches we are constantly searching for breakthroughs. What this book did for me was to reaffirm and confirm where my reading and research have been leading me. Breakthroughs are there right in front of us, we just need to put things in historical context and recombine people, ideas and objects. Breakthrough innovation occurs by fully exploiting the past—looking back to move forward.

Networking is an essential element in achieving breakthroughs; lone rangers seldom achieve breakthrough ideas. Breakthroughs are also the result of getting the right knowledge in the right hands at the correct time; it is amazing to watch what happens when you do that. Formal education in an area can serve as a constraint; Hargadon feels it can force people to conform to the confines of a particular discipline. To achieve breakthroughs start each project with a clean slate. He recommends starting "stupid."

The following quote from Descartes certainly sums up the spirit of the book: "Each problem that I solved became a rule which served afterwards to solve other problems."

ICE

Here are a couple of thoughts from some of my training with Venice Volleyball. Everyday the emphasis is on ICE. What is ICE? It is an acronym for Intensity, Concentration and Effort. That is the way we want the athletes to approach each training session. Of course, those are just empty words if ICE is not stressed and practiced. I try to point out great concentration, effort or intensity and I also remind them when it is not there. We are asking for this for just an hour. This prepares them for the game.

The other thought is that we are seeking 100 percent improvement. Impossible, you say. Well, not really. Think of it this way: If you can improve one percent a day, it is possible or even one percent a week. It is possible but it demands ICE + focus.

Reconditioning

Reconditioning is defined as the period of time that the athlete's emphasis changes from a total focus on therapy to a return to play. Therapists often refer to this period as the gray area; I personally think a better term might be the dark hole. This is the period of time when there seems to be considerable confusion about what the athlete should do, how much, how often and when. It seems that there are two approaches. One way says the athlete is never ready to return to play, so they are stuck in a time warp; the other—the tough guy approach— dumps the athlete immediately back into competition. Obviously there are huge flaws with both.

Here is a method that has worked well for me over the years. First, the reconditioning phase is divided into two sub-phases. The first sub-phase is the return to training. The second sub-phase is the return to the game. The key to success in all of this is that it is *not* protocol driven, it is criteria driven. By that I mean there are tasks or milestones that the athlete must achieve before moving on to the next segment of the program. A protocol is time-based. In essence, it is like social promotion in school—after one week the athlete is magically ready to move to the next step and the next step and so on. This is flawed because everyone progresses at different rates. Some athletes are fast adapters and others are slow adapters; some were at a higher fitness or skill level before they got hurt. All of this demands an individual plan for each athlete that has criteria defined for progress to the next level.

A good starting point is the base level testing data that was taken before the athlete was hurt. Those scores on tests like the 30-second cones jump, agility, or a sprint all represent the 100-percent score that the athlete is capable of. It is unrealistic to expect the athlete to return to 100 percent on all tests. I think they should be at the 90-percent level before being returned to play.

Over the years I have worked out criteria steps that the athlete must achieve in different sports that allow them to gradually return completely into practice. Once they are able to fully practice for an agreed upon time by all those involved then, and only then, are they returned to play. At that point, if it is a team sport and they are a starter, they must be available to return to playing the full time they were playing before injury. I have found gradually phasing them into games makes the psychological transition that much tougher. For this to work there must be flawless communication among all concerned. Above all, the athlete must be an active participant with good feedback. Be sure to video as much as possible to document the criteria skills as they are achieved. This may seem time consuming and to a certain extent it is, but this will ensure that the athlete is 100-percent ready to go with the chance of re-injury minimized.

Prehab

If I hear the term prehab one more time ... What is prehab? It is a term that has no real meaning. I take it as a negative term—to me it means you are preparing to get hurt, because it is inevitable.

I prefer the term remedial work; it is a term I have used for years to describe the injury prevention component of training. It is usually just that—very remedial work designed to address specific individual deficiencies that must be addressed daily to keep the athlete training at optimum efficiency.

Each training session has remedial components that precede the workout and are threaded throughout. It addition, if necessary, the athlete is given remedial *homework*. This may be semantic, but we are talking about very important semantics. Words create images and images create action. You cannot do higher math without the multiplication tables; you cannot write words until you know the alphabet; you cannot perform high-level training activities without remedial work. Lastly, everyone does not have to do the same exercises; remedial work is individually prescribed whenever possible.

Sustained Excellence

One week I had lunch with Jim Steen, Kenyon College Head Swim Coach, who has led Kenyon teams to 29 of 31 NCAA Division III men's championships and 21 of 23 with the women. The conversation with Jim got me thinking again about sustained excellence. The phenomenon of sustained excellence has been something that has interested me for years. I have been fascinated with teams and individuals who can consistently produce at a high level. A lot of this thought was crystallized for me by the book *In Search of Excellence* by Tom Peters. The books *Built to Last* and the classic, *Good to Great* by Jim Collins, certainly identify the characteristics of sustained excellence in business.

I have found that the principles they identified transcend business. The longer I coach and the longer I study this phenomenon, it is clear to me that many are called and few are chosen. Many coaches and athletes just cannot be bothered to do what it takes to achieve at the highest level. It is much easier to talk about being great than it is to be great.

I have chosen some examples from my observations and research. A couple of these teams I have been able to observe first hand, others from afar. I am sure there are other examples but these are the teams that fit my conception of sustained excellence. All are athlete centered, coach driven and administratively supported. The coaches involved live it—they are not about talk and bluster, and they are results oriented. They set a high level of expectation and exceed it through a strong year-round commitment. They think big picture; one play or one game does not a season make. Work ethic is given. Perspective—well, frankly this varies. Some have done better jobs balancing their lives than others.

Talent identification and development is essential. Without talent, excellence is tough to achieve, but some of it is recognizing unique talent and nurturing that. The need for innovation and change are recognized while still maintaining a strong sense of tradition. There is a definite system. If you walked into a UCLA basketball practice when John Wooden was the coach, you saw the system from the first step until the last step. Perhaps the most unifying constant is consistent and continuous leadership. Each of these programs has a strong underlying philosophy that serves as the guiding light.

These are the teams and coaches I have studied. I believe to be excellent you must study excellence and emulate those aspects of excellence that fit your personality or situation.

North Carolina Women's Soccer—Coach Anson Dorrance.
Hard work, dedication and a consistent philosophy are characteristic of this program.

Australian Women's Field Hockey from the 1990's—Coach Ric Charlesworth.
Gold medals in the 1996 and 2000 Olympics plus some world championships thrown in. I was privileged to hear Ric speak in '96 and then meet him. He is dynamic and sets an example that the athletes must be inspired by.

De La Salle High School Football—Coach Bob Ladouceur.
They hold the record for most consecutive wins. They seek out and take on the best, often beating teams that outweigh them by 20 pounds per player. He has a real system that just keeps producing.

Kenyon College Swimming—Coach Jim Steen.
When I worked with Kenyon, I got to see this program first hand. Until recently, when they moved into a new aquatic complex, they trained in a six-lane 25-yard pool! Jim is a real motivator and communicator who sets a high level of expectation.

New England Patriots—Coach Bill Belichick.
A system that works in pro sports, he demands practice effort—almost unheard of in this world of high-paid prima donnas.

Adams State College Cross Country—Coach Joe Vigil.

Joe is one of my mentors. When he coached at Adams State they were unbeatable. He took local Colorado kids that no one else wanted and turned them into champions.

UCLA Basketball—Coach John Wooden.

In my book, this man and his program set the example for all to follow.

Saint Johns University (Minnesota)—John Gagliardi.

He is the most non-traditional football coach ever! They do not scrimmage, they do not hit in practice, they do not study film, they have no formal off-season conditioning program. Despite this, or actually because of this, they go deep into the DIII playoffs each year. John Gagliardi is still coaching into his early-80s and he began coaching his high school team when he was 16! That is longevity and sustained excellence.

Homework

Have you done your homework? I was watching a program on CNBC the other night called *Mad Money* with Jim Cramer. It is certainly not something I watch with regularity, but I had read an interview with him that I found quite interesting. The investing part was interesting, but the coaching implications were even more interesting to me. His big thing is homework. He recommends an hour of research homework for every stock you own. I started thinking, and that is what the good coaches I know do. Before they go out to the field or the track they really do their homework. Each segment, each exercise is planned. When the workout is over they evaluate the workout in the context of the whole plan. There are no knee-jerk responses; they are disciplined, just like a good investor. I know I can spend up to three hours a week planning for the subsequent week. Each workout takes about 15 to 20 minutes of planning. This work up front pays rich dividends, and there are few surprises. Progress is predictable and steady; conversely, lack of progress is explainable and easily corrected. Make sure you do your homework.

Relevance

Is what you are doing relevant? Last night I was reading a book called *FutureThink*, by Edie Weiner and Arnold Brown, and there was an anecdote in there that made me think about relevance, as well as tradition and resistance to change. An American officer was observing a British artillery battery training on maneuvers, just before WWII. He noticed that the battery had seven men. Six men were fully engaged in activity and the seventh man stood at attention the whole time. The American officer asked his British counterpart what he was doing and he answered that he did not know why he was standing at attention but he would find out. The next day he told the American officer that he had had found out and that the seventh man had held the horses! Are you standing at attention waiting for the horses?

A Few Good People

I am writing this post in reaction to what I am seeing today in the field. We have more certifications that ever before, more educational programs and resources than ever, and yet we have fewer people qualified to be athletic development coaches. How is that possible? The problem is that there are not enough people who have experience, or worked to gain the experience, of hands-on, down and dirty coaching. I do not mean supervising a weight room or personal training. I mean putting together a whole program that incorporates all components of athletic performance. Being responsible for your athlete's performance in the game, meet or match, having to take ownership and put yourself on the line. I run into more book smart young men and women today who think they are qualified to coach at the highest levels and yet they have *never* coached. Let's get real here. I am looking for a few good people who have coaching experience—I mean real coaching, like little league, Pop Warner, or any situation where you must organize and teach A to Z—who also have the education and want to learn, grow and define the profession. I am going to post more specific criteria on the Web site next week. There will be jobs for you. You must be dynamic and passionate and willing to work for peanuts. You must be willing to pay your dues. You have to live it. I am working to create jobs for people, but I cannot find enough people who are committed and willing to pay their dues to fill the jobs.

Injuries in Football

I am not privy to the daily injury reports of any NFL team, so I only see what everyone sees in the popular press, but my perception is that preventable injuries are not declining. For me, preventable injuries are muscle pulls. I even think some non-contact ankle sprains and knee sprains can, at the very least, be minimized. Our local paper recently implored Jon Gruden, the coach of the Tampa Bay Buccaneers, to look into why they have had so many injuries. I do not know who the strength coach is there, and I have no idea what their program consists of, but the article made me think.

Here are a few of my thoughts: Today, every NFL team has a strength coach and in most cases an assistant, but how many are allowed to do their job? How many of them really concern themselves with injury prevention? How many of the injuries are caused by the type of strength training they employ? What do they do to warm up for practices and games? How many of their players employ personal trainers who have a different agenda than the club that pays the players' salary? Just some food for thought.

Injuries in Pro Sports

Someone wrote in with this comment:

> The other thing that you always have to consider with the NFL is so many of these guys have "specialists" they see all over the place during the season and during the off-season. Everyone seems to have a specialist or guru they depend on to get through.

This is a major cause of the problem. It is true in basketball and baseball too. These people have no accountability to the teams that pay the players. They are not in the loop with the team trainers, the conditioning coach or anyone else associated with the team. Incidentally, it was these *specialists* who were also the source of the drug problem in baseball—look at Barry Bonds' trainer, or the problems they had with the Texas Rangers. From what I have seen, their agenda is to please the player and not do what is necessary to ensure that the player will stay healthy. They are not at practice, so they have no idea what the player did before they arrived. If they are medical people they duplicate treatment or prescribe contradictory treatment.

Who is to blame for this? I put the blame right in the lap of the teams. They are letting the inmates run the prison. They are afraid of the agents and the player's associations. I fought this battle with a team I worked with—basically, they were afraid of the agents and did not want to anger a player. Yet, now the teams are holding team conditioning and medical personnel accountable for something they may not have control over.

Also, another problem that is the fault of the teams is bidding out medical services to the highest bidder. That does not ensure the best medical care, it merely compensates someone who has marketed themselves well. Same thing with conditioning staff. They have no idea what is good and bad. If they see a lot of activity they think that is good. Folks, I have seen all of this—doctors who were incompetent, conditioning coaches handing out programs that were terrible! All of this plays into the hands of the agents and the players because then they go looking for something better. The more I look back on my nine years with the White Sox, the more I realize that we were able to do it right, but that was another era.

Another Year Coaching

It seems like just yesterday that I walked out of the field house in January, 1969, at Santa Barbara High School, to be greeted by 85 eager 10th, 11th and 12th graders all identically dressed in gym uniforms (boy, is it different now). This was still the first semester, but under CIF rules, you could begin track practice during the athletic period.

When the second semester started and basketball was over, the number swelled to 130. Santa Barbara High had a great tradition in track and field. Over the years it had produced numerous California State champions and place winners. Little did I know that cool January day, that in June I would be privileged to coach their next state champion. The head coach was Bill Crow. There are not enough superlatives to describe this man and the opportunity he gave me. By the end of his career, Bill had won over 160 meets while losing only 24—an incredible record. Bill was one of the toughest, most demanding individuals I have known, but in a very quiet way. He was a man small in stature, maybe 5'6", but he commanded respect. He would stand on the judges' stand with a megaphone and you had better be ready when he called you.

In 1975, when Bill retired, I was chosen to be the next coach at Santa Barbara High School. Needless to say it was a privilege and an honor to try to fill Bill's shoes. There was no way I was going to replace him. It was like taking over from John Wooden. My goal throughout my career has been to be half as good a coach as Bill. Basically, for those three weeks in 1969 before the second semester started he turned the team over to me to condition them. He told me I would be coaching the shot putters and the jumpers, but not the pole vault. The coach of the vaulters was Gates Foss, a retired volunteer, and another coaching legend. It seemed that every year Gates had a 14-foot vaulter. No matter if they were big or small, fast or slow, Gates seemed to turn them out.

As I reflect on that experience and the tremendous start it gave me, I am excited to move forward and begin the next year coaching. Unfortunately, I will not be coaching track and field, my first love, but I will be getting the opportunity to work with some great coaches and kids who are eager to improve.

Looking Back to Move Ahead

I just finished a 90-minute ride to start the New Year off on a good foot. During that ride I was thinking about this blog and continuing to reflect on the past few years, which have been years of change, renewal, reinvention and discovery.

In 2005, when I left my job working with the Nike Oregon Project, I had to move on and find my way quickly. I decided to finish the book which I had worked on in fits and starts for the previous three years. I figured that would get me back on track and reignite my passion for coaching and learning.

As I was driving back home to Florida I had a lot of time to think and reflect. I was in the middle of Wyoming when I got the idea of the *functional path*. I came to the conclusion that trying to follow the functional path was what it was all about. I felt that if I was struggling to stay on the functional path then others must be doing the same. That is where this blog started. I had to wait for my son to come home from India before launching it because it was technologically beyond my capabilities.

I have found the blog to be a great starting point for the day. It is certainly a forum, and it is a responsibility I do not take lightly. It is part of my mission to move forward and define the field of athletic enhancement. My goal is to be a voice of reason and a source of basic knowledge. I struggle at times to strike a balance between sharing and educating and the marketing necessary to make a living. I try to stay away from hype; I will leave that to the gurus.

Every year between Christmas and the New Year, I use the week as a think week—a week to reflect, study, renew, catch up and think big thoughts. Here are some thoughts, lessons and ideas. Some are old ideas that have been reinforced, some are new and some may not seem especially profound to anyone but me:

- Respect is earned not bought.

- Knowledge and wisdom eventually win out over hype and promotion.

- Coaching is special because of the impact you can have on lives and the daily lessons you learn.

• I am an idealist. I dream of the way things should be and try to make them happen.

• Knowledge without passion is wasted; people do their best when they are passionately engaged.

• There is no set formula for training; there are principles that are highly adaptive.

• Understanding context is essential.

• Many new ideas are just old ideas repackaged.

• I specialize in being a generalist.

• Research and science are wonderful, but they must be tempered with practice and common sense.

• Coaching is talking, listening, seeing and doing. It is totally multi-dimensional. It is not about me, it is about we and us.

• Friendship is special; cherish your friends.

• Family is even more special; they must be first and foremost.

• Make every experience you have a one-off experience; make what you do each day special. If you don't approach it that way, the people you work with won't either.

• Don't make resolutions or set goals. Instead, go out and do something, take action; don't set goals, achieve them!

Solving Movement Problems

A reader wrote:

> In your book, Athletic Development, *you have a wonderful chapter on Movement Aptitude and Balance. Can you describe some of your strategies for teaching movement awareness? On page 146, you say to give athletes movement problems to solve that will enable them to discover movement skills. Can you give some examples of this? Thanks for your book, it is great!*

It is pretty simple actually. For example, you tell the person that they have to get from point A to point B as fast as possible. Put out three obstacles that they must traverse that prevent them from going from A to B. Let them figure it out. They may have to climb over one obstacle, crawl under another and jump over something. Let them figure it out and then when they are finished, debrief them and ask them why they did what they did. If you want to add pressure, then add a time element.

Make it a game. With kids, have them imitate animals. Make it reflexive, not cognitive. Playful is best; make it *FUNdamental,* and believe me they will figure it out.

Approaching Sixty and Training

A reader posted this:

> There are a lot of us approaching 60, and your blog recounts issues that most of us are facing. Your books are excellent for younger athletes—how about a paper or a book on using your techniques focusing on fitness for those of us "approaching 60?"

I am fast approaching 60, with only a little over two weeks to go, so this is an area near to my heart. Here are some thoughts on things I have personally observed as well as what I have been able to pull from research.

Less is more—in fact, much less is a lot more. Train consistently but remember that training is cumulative. If you have been an athlete, like I was, and have continued to workout there is an accumulation of background. I have found that shorter, more intense workouts are preferable to more prolonged workouts. Follow these workouts by a much lighter day. If it is a higher impact day then follow it with a very low impact day. I know I get in trouble when I try to put two impact workouts back-to-back.

Just as training is cumulative, the old injuries are still there. Respect your injury history and do more remedial type of work so they do not come back to haunt you.

Warm up, which is even more important as you age. Make it active and progressive. Be sure to include rotational movements and some crawling. Ninety percent of the warm-up should be on your feet and moving at no slower than a jog tempo.

Don't buy into the aerobics myth. Don't get me wrong, you must do aerobic work, but it should be balanced by all the other components of training. Strength training, especially exercises that promote postural integrity and dynamic alignment, must be done consistently. Vary your mode of aerobic work and don't be afraid to push it a bit.

Flexibility is more important. Aging is relentless, but it seems the most relentless is the loss of range of motion. I must admit I have been very flexible all my life, but in the last year I have noticed some subtle losses in flexibility. I must make a conscious effort to incorporate this component daily. Yoga is good, especially Ashtanga yoga. Hip mobility is really essential. I prefer hurdle walks to achieve this, because it is dynamic and I have a consistent measure.

Balance—train it in a sensible manner. Make it part of other activities and be as dynamic as possible.

Agility work is very important. You don't have to do bag drills from your football days, but body awareness work and some movements that involve quick changes of direction and reorientation of the body should be done twice a week, even if you are an endurance athlete.

Last but not least, aging is relentless. There is no fountain of youth, but exercise and an athletic lifestyle come close. You are only as old as you think you are. I live in a community of newlyweds and nearly-deads. It looks like a snapshot of the future of the U.S. with a population that's primarily over 55. I am inspired daily by the people in their sixth, seventh and eighth decades of life and how active and athletic they are. When I go swim there is an 80-year-old man who has had a triple bypass who swims a mile a day. When you talk to him he doesn't talk like he is old and he doesn't act it. My motto is: older and better. My goal is to die doing a smorgy circuit with the breakfast club when I am in my 90s.

No Step Back

I have read the study that is the basis of the so-called *plyo step* and I do not come to the same profound conclusions. In fact, I have read it three times just in case I missed something. The opening sentence in the introduction is a giveaway to me: "In most types of sport the human body must accelerate from a stationary position to maximal speed." In fact, in the majority of sports, starts are moving and involve movement in multiple directions. Later in the introduction the following sentence appears: "In starting from the standing position it is noteworthy that first the push-off leg is placed backward." In fact, the push-off leg, the leg that is in contact with the ground the longest, is forward and the so-called *fast leg*, the leg that moves first, is placed back.

As I evaluate the study, their conclusions regarding the paradoxical step are true, given the narrow starting conditions that they define. They found what they were looking for. Look carefully at the research design. They did not really try different starting techniques, and they were very narrow in their selection. Standing tall with the feet in close proximity hardly ever occurs in sport. My conclusion is that if you want to execute a fast first step and that is all that matters, then step back, but make sure you are in a tall position with the feet together.

The other problem I have with the study is that they just looked at the first step. The first step is just a means to commence acceleration. To truly assess any starting technique you must look at what happens at five, ten and even twenty meters. Franklin Henry, eons ago in his seminal work on the sprint start, showed that the bunch start was the fastest start but did not result in the fastest time at the finish. The starting position and first step must be put in context.

In conclusion, looking at research is great, but it must be carefully evaluated in the context of what happens in the real world. You cannot draw profound general conclusions from one narrowly defined study. I spend about 20 percent of my week studying and evaluating research and I always have to remind myself of this. I suggest that those of you who are interested in starting, look at the stumble reflex. That is where the answer lies. The bottom line is that in taking a positive step to set acceleration to optimum speed, don't step back!

False Step

A false step is defined as a step that is a step away from the intended direction of movement. Generally, a false step is a wasted step. There are situations where a false step is used to gain a tactical advantage—most specifically, a running back in football will use a false step to gain depth or to time up a handoff. The moral of the story again is always look at movements in context.

The more I have thought about the whole first-step scenario the more I come back to context. The first step is only one part of a bigger picture. What is the purpose of the first step? The purpose of the first step is to displace the center of gravity in the intended direction and create a positive shin angle to effectively apply force back against the ground. I break movement down into the following components:

1. Stance or starting position.
2. Start.

3. First step:
   a. Position.
   b. Direction.
4. Getaway Step (Second Step).
5. Acceleration to optimum speed.
6. Deceleration.
7. Possible reacceleration.
8. Stopping.

This whole scenario takes place in about two to three seconds, possibly four seconds at the maximum. The ultimate goal is to keep each of the segments in the context of the ultimate objective, which is to stop effectively and make the play. It is also to recognize that in the majority of sports, starts are moving, not stationary. This does minimize the importance of the first step and in many ways accentuates the necessity of creating a good shin angle on the first step.

My stance is based on biomechanical research not anecdotal opinion. When I say we researched this with the White Sox, we commissioned Dr. Lois Klatt from Concordia University to do a biomechanical analysis of the three first-step scenarios. One of the scenarios was the false step; it is not more efficient. The first-step action that results in displacement of the center of gravity in the intended direction is far superior. The plyo step gives the perception of a faster movement but it does not result in displacement of the center of gravity in the intended direction.

A false step can be used, as I pointed out, in certain tactical situations, to position the body, gain depth or serve as a deceptive mechanism. Frankly, coaching someone out of the false step is very natural if you correctly place their hip in relation to the base of support. The bottom line is that I want my center of gravity moving in the intended direction as soon as possible.

I have seen the stuff on the so-called *plyo step* to take advantage of the stretch shortening cycle. The problem is that it is not a fair trade off. You gain more with a positive step. We researched this in 1989 looking at base running stance and start. There were three different footwork patterns studied. In short, the positive step gave an advantage that was clear at one, five and ten yards. The two false-step scenarios, one of which could be considered a plyo loading step, resulted in a disadvantage that was never regained.

Gravity Wins!

Gravity always wins. Sometimes you can cheat it, but eventually it will get you. I have been doing an intensive aging and exercise study as I am fast approaching 60. I have been quite focused and dedicated since July, save a few jaunts over the pond, which interrupted my training. The focus has been on re-establishing a good strength base, focusing on the ability to handle my body weight, and a huge core strength emphasis. By and large it has gone well. I still really need to lose at least ten pounds, but that is another kind of discipline I am trying to find.

So the time has come to begin to do more running. So far the focus has been on lower impact stuff like biking and swimming, although we have done a fair bit of agility work.

Saturday was the first running day, and it was great! Fifteen-second runs and fifteen-second walks felt good, with all the moving parts moving. The sensible thing to do, would have been to swim, bike or just do core work on Sunday. Who said common sense is common? I even verbalized to Mike Lane, my friend who was training with me, how it would be best if we only warmed up and didn't run too much. That would be too easy. We both had very tight hamstrings so we warmed up well and did some jog, skip, run progressions and then did circle runs (my theory is that that works the lateral hamstring— that is another story). I felt something in my hip. I ignored it and stretched it. It got stiffer as the day went on. Wait, it gets better.

So we met midday Monday for a workout. We did a hood warm-up: a bit of ABC Ladder and the DB PPS Squat workout, plus a 100-meter run after each complex. Bam, the hip went, but of course I finished the workout. Then I went for a twenty-minute swim. It felt good after that but as the day went on it stiffened up even more. Now I am crawling up the stairs. I will probably not be able to workout today and I am supposed to know what I am doing. Gravity will always win!

The moral of this painful tale of stupidity is, if in doubt, do less. Where is the ASTYM when I need it?

Timing

I love to body surf and that is what made me think of timing. During the summer when there were storms off Baja, California and the surf was up, we would spend hours body surfing. When you caught the wave just right it was a great ride. You could ride those big ones right into the beach. If you were late getting into the wave sometimes the wave just passed under you and occasionally you got dumped. If you were too early, that was a disaster. You got caught in the wave and it was like being inside a washing machine. Then there were days when everything clicked—every wave was perfect and your timing was right on.

Timing is everything—how many times have you heard that one? In training, nothing could be truer. Sometimes it is not necessarily what you do, but when you do it. The correct workout or exercise done at the wrong time can spell disaster for a training program. It is about why you are doing what you are doing and when you are doing it. Next time you are thinking about workout design, picture yourself in the water catching a wave. Time it so that you ride that wave to the beach.

Coaching the Monster Age Group

One of the toughest age groups to coach is the 12-to-15 age group. I call it the *monster age group*. This is probably the most uncomfortable time of their lives. The boys may or may not have gone through puberty; most likely the girls have. Therefore, the girls are more physically developed, but very embarrassed about it. They can beat the boys, but probably do not want to, because they want the boys to ask them to the dance. Who wants to go to a dance with someone who kicked your butt in the pool or on the track? The boys make up for all of this by being obnoxious and acting stupid to cover up all of their insecurities.

Obviously, from a coaching perspective there are huge psycho, social and physical development issues that appear with this age group that are unique. Coaches of this age group must be prepared to deal with these issues. This is a good time to train boys and girls separately. Girls who have gone through puberty need to be pushed in training a bit more, especially in regard to strength training. Boys at this age are better off in groups where they are not singled out. Because of the growth spurt that occurs, here the work must emphasize control of their body and body awareness. Be careful about ignoring the slow developer, they will come on like gangbusters later on. As a coach of this *monster age group* the rewards are many; you will see changes faster than at any other age. You will see boys become men and girls become women. Remember, it is a painful process for them, so don't expect it to be easy for you.

Moneyball Myth

If any of you have read the book *Moneyball* by Michael Lewis, it certainly has an appeal. It seems that innovation has come to a traditional sport like baseball. Folks, I will break it to you slowly, moneyball is all a myth. It is about money, but it is the indiscriminate use of dollars on questionable oft-injured players. If you applied the moneyball formula to most of the free agent signings that have occurred recently almost all the players would be looking for a real job. Lest we forget, this is not about sport, it is about entertainment. One simple solution is non-guaranteed contracts like the NFL.

Factors to Consider When Developing a Plan

- Demands of the event or position.
- Qualities of the individual athlete.
- Pattern of injuries/injury history.

- "24-Hour Athlete" concept.
- Gender.
- The time frame available to execute the plan.
- Specific goals.
- Developmental level:
    Current state of fitness.
- Current technical development.
- Competitive Schedule:
    Qualifying Format.
- Championship format.
- Recovery/Regeneration.

The Planning Process

The long-term plan is a general guide. The long-term plan is still organized in the traditional manner with phases or blocks, with training components divided into major and minor emphases. The following is an example from soccer:

The individual training session is the cornerstone of the entire training plan. The individual training session is where the long-term plan is actually implemented.

A long-term plan is a succession of linked, individual training sessions in pursuit of specific objectives.

The training session should occupy the greatest emphasis in planning and execution.

Each session must be carefully evaluated and the following sessions adjusted accordingly.

Contingency planning is a very important and a necessary part of the long-term planning process. It is especially important to have contingency plans ready for individual training sessions.

Planning the Session

Each training session should a have general theme.

This general theme, in turn, should be supported by objectives for each component in that training session that are very specific and measurable.

When planning an individual training session, ask yourself, what do I most need to accomplish? How does that session fit into the bigger picture? Carefully consider the time available for training and recovery.

Every component in the workout must be in pursuit of the specific objectives of the workout and follow the general theme for that particular session.

The workout is not an end in itself; it is, however, a means to an end. Therefore, it must be put in the context of the whole training plan, so it is important to not let the individual training session get blown out of proportion.

The key is to design the sessions so that there is a seamless flow from one workout into another, so that even though the focus is on that individual workout, it always must be placed in the context of the workout leading into and out of it.

The actual design of the session should carefully consider:

- Progression/Sequence.
- Training time available and time allocation.
- Integration with skill workouts.
- Size of the facility or training area relative to the number of athletes training.
- Equipment available.
- Coaching personnel available as well as the number of athletes that will participate in the actual training session.

Remedial Component

Make sure that there is always an injury prevention component in each workout. This is most easily addressed in the warm-up. Given the constraints of most situations, special consideration needs to be given to recovery and how to incorporate it. Self-massage, shaking and stretching as well as intra-workout nutrition in the form of hydration is the most basic and practical form of intra-workout recovery.

Team or Group Training

When training a group, carefully plan to meet individual needs in a group context. Everyone will not progress and learn at the same rate.

Multiple Workouts

Multiple workouts in a day allow the workouts to be even more focused and shorter in duration. Multiple sessions are a necessity for the elite athlete.

Training Effects

The physiological, biomechanical, or psychological changes that occur when training are:

- Acute—Changes that occur during the training session.
- Immediate—Changes that occur from one single workout or a training day.
- Cumulative (Delayed Training Effect)—Changes that occur from a series of workouts.
- Delayed—Changes over time from a specific training program.
- Residual—Changes that are retained after training that quality is discontinued.

Remember, no one workout can make an athlete, but one workout can break an athlete, therefore, the focus should be on the accumulation of the training effects. It is imperative to carefully plan the sequence of training sessions from day-to-day and within the day, as well as project the potential effect of training on subsequent days. With this in mind, always be aware of the residual training effect. The ultimate goal is the cumulative training effect, which is what occurs in the long-term. Where does the workout fit within the microcycle plan? The workout is only one component of the big picture.

Complimentary Training Units

To achieve positive training adaptations look carefully at complementary components both intra- and inter-workouts. Complementary training units are components that work together to enhance each other. The traditional approach has been to consider this intra-workout, but it is also important to consider inter-workout, both between sessions in a day and between days. Examples of complimentary training units are:

- Speed and Strength.
- Strength and Elastic Strength.
- Endurance and Strength Endurance.
- Skill, Speed and Elastic Strength.

Ultimately, the units have more than a complementary relationship. They should enhance each other and mesh, with the ultimate effect being synergistic. The simplest means to address the complementary nature of training is to utilize the modular training approach.

Training Modules

The basis of planning the individual training session is the modular training concept. This will make planning and implementation of workouts very easy, as well as address the need for complementary training components both intra- and inter-workout.

The training module consists of specific combinations and sequences of exercises that are designed to be very specific and compatible. The exercises are carefully selected to sequence and flow from one exercise to the next within the module. Each module is designed to focus on one particular component that should fit with the other modules in that training session. The volume and intensity for the exercises within each module is determined for each session based on analysis of the previous session. A training session is a collection of modules.

Injuries Caused by Training

I am hearing more and more reports from colleagues who are ATCs and physical therapists about injuries caused by training. Some of the stories are, frankly, borderline negligent. This is something that really concerns me, because it is a negative reflection on all of us in the field. Improper workout design, inappropriate exercise selection and failure to communicate with the coaches is inexcusable. The most recent incident I've heard of occurred in volleyball at a major DI (drill instructor) school. The strength coach had his own agenda. He was not listening to the coaches, and had no regard for the demands of practice and the competition schedule. The result was a rash of shoulder injuries. At the same school, two days before the start of two-a-day practices, the football players were tested on 1RM squats and the punter hurt his back and was unable to practice for five days. Why test in that close a proximity to two-a-days and why max test a punter?

These are the kinds of things I keep hearing over and over. I know you have to be careful when you paint with a broad brush stroke and sound like you are pointing fingers. That is not my intention. My intention is to call attention to a growing problem. We must more clearly define the field. We need to do a better job training athletic development coaches. More certifications are not the answer. We must have hands-on training of coaches. Strength coaches need to become athletic development coaches and get out of the weight room, which is only one piece of the puzzle. At times, it is a big piece of the puzzle in certain sports and at certain times of the training year. We must be involved with all aspects of the athlete's life.

When is There Enough?

We certainly do live in a culture of excess, but do we have to go over the top with our young, developing high school athletes? Have we taken the focus away from interscholastic competition and shifted it to commercially-sponsored, elite all-star games, national championships and showcase camps? It seems that what we are doing is trying to find the best earlier, instead of a more egalitarian approach of getting more kids involved and keeping them involved.

There was a saying I remember my parents using when I was growing up, "How do you keep them down on the farm after they have seen Paris?" A normal high school game has become mundane. It seems it must be televised and hyped to the max or it does not have worth.That's rubbish. Let's let the kids be kids. Take all that money used to hype and promote all of those all-star games and camps and invest in getting more kids involved and raise the standard of coaching. It should be about promoting sport and better coaching.

Design Thinking and Coaching

Everything old is new again. Every time I do anything or talk to anyone, no matter what the field, it seems this statement comes up. During the recent past I have been focusing my reading and research on design and innovation. The more I read about design and innovation, the truer the adage becomes.

Obviously, to innovate you have to start somewhere. It seems that for those who are most innovative the best place to start is on a path that someone else has traveled. Innovation demands a blurring of the boundaries between sports and various disciplines that contribute to sport performance. Here is the announcement of a new class at the Stanford University Design School that reinforces that idea:

Immersive experiences in innovation and design thinking, blurring the boundaries between technology, business, and human values. Explore the tenets of design thinking including being human-centered, prototype driven and mindful of process in everything you do.

This really resonated with me, especially the last part.

Coaching is human-centered. It is prototype driven; we are always prototyping, and it is a very mindful process. This is what coaching really should be. Design thinking offers the coaching profession a fresh look at old ideas and the ability to take those ideas and innovate.

Drills

To drill or not to drill? That is the question. During my coaching career, I have seen the pendulum swing several times on this issue. I have seen periods where the trend was to break everything down into its smallest parts and then drill those parts, and hope that the drills would positively affect the whole action. I have also seen times where the emphasis was on the whole action with a minimum of drill work. Today, from my perspective, it appears we are in another drill era. That is fine as long as it is not carried too far. The drills must not become an end unto themselves; they must be a means to an end.

Before designing drills make sure that you completely understand the whole action. Always relate the drill back to the whole action. Try to distinguish similar and same. Think whole/part/whole. Mastery of a drill does not necessarily mean that the drill will transfer to the whole. It has been my experience that too much drill work ultimately ends up with the whole action being very segmented and choppy. I also think beginners should not be taught too many drills. They should get a feel for the whole and explore the whole movement before beginning to break it down into parts.

I have seen this over and over in soccer. Young players are taught a plethora of fancy drills with no idea of how those drills flow into a game. They are also taught these drills before they are physically mature enough to get a good feel for them. Rather than spending time on drills, we should allow practices to be more playful and game-like.

Another example of drills run amok are sprint drills. Instead, teach someone a feel for running fast by playing task-oriented games that make them feel different rhythms and stride patterns. Making it game-like removes the skill from the cognitive domain and they learn by discovery. I know at this time you are probably thinking, what about the mistakes they are making? Learn from mistakes. Contrast what feels good and what feels bad. Drills can have a place, but think about the ultimate objective. A seasoned performer who is working to perfect a small technical error will, in all probability, benefit more from drills than a rank beginner.

Finally, apply this check list before you use a drill:
- What is the drill?
- Why use the drill?
- How is it executed?
- When would it be used?
- Does the athlete relate to it?

If you have good answers for all of these then go for it!

Philosophy Regarding Workouts

I am very guarded about sending out workouts. This is not because they are full of secrets, or because I am trying to be a guru who sells everything he does. It is more about my basic philosophy. The workouts that I make up are usually for a specific person, or for a specific team. I've worked with them—I know the training age, and level of development. I know any physical limitations they might have. I will either administer the workout myself or have someone I have trained administer the workout.

My experience has shown that people copy the workouts and use them with athletes or teams that are inappropriate for the workout design. The result is that people do not improve or even worse, they get hurt.

The old cliché that applies here is you can feed a man a fish or you can teach him how to fish. I would prefer to teach him how to fish. I think that is what underlies everything I do. If I work with an athlete for a period of time, he or she should be able to coach themselves. If they cannot, I have not succeeded. I am always trying to work myself out of a job. I work hard to teach them why they are doing what they are doing. It is always more than an exercise; it is how the workout fits into the context of the whole training program. Those of you who have attended my seminars have learned the why, and in certain seminars, the how.

Workout Design Insights

"I cannot teach anybody anything; I can only make them think." —Socrates.

A much greater mind than mine sums up the philosophy. I am going to work harder to make all of you think. There is no real secret to workout design. The answer is right in front of you. Look at the sport you are working with, thoroughly understand it, do not make any assumptions, know the athletes strengths and weaknesses, have a clear objective and a plan to execute the objective and go for it!

Training Young Runners

Yes, you are what you train to be, so the first mistake people make in training young runners, or swimmers for that matter, is to pile on the miles. Build that big aerobic base and get them really slow. It is preferable to start with good, sound running mechanics and get them comfortable running fast. Then gradually build up their ability to carry that speed. That does not mean to imply that it is an either/or proposition, but it should be a mix or a blend.

The reason the U.S. is struggling to produce distance runners is that during the prime years when speed can be developed, they are out slogging on the roads, learning how to run slow and getting rewarded for it. In 1972, we had five boys, ninth-graders, run from 4:50 down to 4:30 in the mile. None of those boys ran over five miles in any one run, they never ran twice a day and peak mileage was 30 miles for one of the boys. All the rest were around 25 miles. They were all good athletes; they had five days a week of vigorous physical education. They had fun and played other sports.

It is not rocket science; it is common sense. Treat the runner like an athlete. Get them functionally fit and make sure they get familiar with all three planes of motion. If you do that, they won't get hurt; they will get faster and they will have a great experience. Remember, keep it *FUNdamental*.

You Are What You Train to Be

You are what you train to be. I was taught that valuable lesson in a great class I had at UCSB in 1969 called Fundamentals of Conditioning, taught by Sherm Button. I have forgotten a lot of things from the class but I never have forgotten that lesson. If you train to be slow you will be slow; if you train to be fast you will be fast. Sounds simple, and it is, but simplicity yields complexity. It is the simple axioms like this that are easy to forget.

Frankly, that is why when I look at some of the strength training programs that are the current rage, and wonder where common sense enters into the picture. Doing everything with chains and bands and box squatting may make you measurably stronger, but does doing those slow movements all the time transfer? Based on what I learned a long time ago, I don't think so. Do those modes of training have a place? Sure they do, at certain phases, in small quantities to vary stimulus, but a steady diet will not improve explosive power. It all comes down to keeping a clear focus on what you are training for. Look carefully at the physical qualities demanded and train those qualities. You can get away with goofy stuff for a while, but eventually it will come back to haunt you.

I remember a defensive back from here in Sarasota who went to an SEC (Southeastern Conference) school and started for four years. At the end of his senior season when he had to improve his 40 time, I was talking to him. I had just watched him run and he ran like he was pulling a heavy sled. I asked him what they had done at his school. Lo and behold, they had done repeat 100-yard sled pulls with up to 200 pounds. No wonder he ran like he was pulling a sled—that was what was ingrained in his nervous system. Remember the message, you are what you train to be.

There is a line from a country and western song that sums it up quite well: "Work your fingers to the bone, what do you get? Boney fingers!"

Pressure

I spent Saturday afternoon and evening doing something I have not done in a very long time— I actually watched football games. Usually, within three minutes I am asleep and the game is watching me. I watched the USC versus UCLA game, a historic rivalry, rich in tradition, but the stakes were higher this time: A berth in the national championship game for USC if they won.

The reason I watched the football games and also watched parts of the men's and women's NCAA soccer championships is that I am fascinated with how athletes and coaches deal with big game pressure. Getting there is one thing, but achieving optimum performance in the big game is another. It was obvious from the start that USC was feeling the pressure; the false start penalties by their linemen were an indicator of that. I also wonder if they had played to win too often; too many must-win games can be an emotional drain.

On the other hand, watching Florida versus Arkansas in the SEC championship game was like watching a team going to work. Florida made mistakes, but they had a resiliency and focus that was relentless. It was interesting to watch their coach Urban Meyer. This guy is driven and intense and his team reflects him. When the players dumped Gatorade on him and there was still 50 seconds left in the game, he was annoyed; he clearly sent a message to his players that the game was not over until the final whistle.

Over the years, I have seen athletes and coaches fail and succeed. One of the biggest characteristics of those who fail is that they feel it is the big game and they have to do something different. A wise cowboy once said, "Dance with who brung you." In other words, do the things that got you there when you are there.

I love to watch Tom Brady. He loves the pressure and he is best under pressure. That is also why it was so much fun to watch Joe Montana. The demeanor and the body language never changed and that had a calming effect on his teammates. As a coach I love pressure. I like to be around the atmosphere where excellence is the only option. Have I messed up in pressure situations? Yes, big time, but hopefully I have learned from those mistakes. The secret is having fun. Do the things that got you to the big game, learn what buttons to push with individuals and the team. Most of the time it is not a matter of getting psyched up, it is a matter of staying focused and in the moment. The atmosphere of the big game or the championship is enough to put most people over the top.

The other aspect is to prepare over the long term for the big game. Put the state meet or state championship in the schedule and talk about it all the time. That is the ultimate goal. Make it familiar. Simulate the pressure situations in training as often as possible, not just in technical and tactical situations, but also in strength training, speed development and conditioning. Find out who thrives on pressure, who can make quick decisions, and don't wait until the big game to find out.

It was interesting watching the North Carolina women, as they were actually having fun. One of them got knocked flat on her back, but when her teammates came over to help her up she was laughing. Man, did that send a message to Notre Dame. Her body language said, you gave me your best shot and it wasn't good enough. Why? Because that is the way they practice—they practice to be in the big game all year. Michael Jordon was a tremendous pressure performer because he put pressure on himself and his teammates every day in training. That is as good a way as any to prepare for the pressure.

Isokinetic Testing

It is absolutely amazing to me that people still make extensive use of isokinetic testing for injury screening, rehabilitation and research. This was considered cutting edge in the 1970s when we did not know any better. At best, isokinetic testing serves as a random number generator. It tells us what an individual muscle or group of muscles is capable of in a very controlled (but very unnatural) sterile environment.

In the late '70s and early '80s, at various USOC camps in track and field, we did extensive isokinetic testing, because we felt we needed to assess strength. I remember puzzling over the results of my athletes' test results. The numbers never made sense to me. Sure, there were right-to-left differences, but when I began to understand that the body is fundamentally asymmetrical, that concern was alleviated.

Then there was the infamous hamstring-to-quadriceps ratio. As the speed of testing went up to 300 degrees/sec the hamstring-to-quadriceps ratio became 1:1. What was that telling us? Well, it was telling us what we now know from biomechanical analysis about hamstring function and muscle architecture from the work of Liebert. How about in rehab as an indicator that strength is sufficient to return to play? Absolutely not. I have seen athletes with great isokinetic scores limp out of the therapy clinic. They were ready to play?

In summary, an isolated single joint, single plane test done at speeds no where near performance speeds, in a proprioceptively unchallenging environment tells us virtually nothing about the ability to perform beyond that isolated test.

Evaluating Training Programs

I have received several e-mails asking for comments on various training programs. I always find this difficult. Often when you see a program posted on the Internet in various discussion groups or published in a journal, the workouts are taken out of context. By that I mean you cannot see the phase that preceded the workouts, and often it is not very clear where the workouts are leading. Also important is what population, in terms of developmental age, the workout is aimed at.

Much of the recent discussion on sprint mechanics is a good example of another problem: taking someone else's ideas or research and putting your own twist on it. To combat this, I always try to go straight to the source, personally if possible. I visited with Bosch and Klomp, as well as Peter Weyand. I was involved in Ralph Mann's original research. All of them have been misinterpreted. Read the research and stop and analyze it logically. I still have not met a scientist who innovated a training concept. They follow coaches and verify or refute.

I think it is important to understand that there are no magic training programs. Many times people succeed in spite of, not because of, what they do. I also know that there is often a big difference between what athletes or coaches say they do in training and what they actually do. I have observed that phenomenon first hand many times. Once again use common sense, and think about what the "experts" are saying.

Remember another key point. Training is more than getting tired. Anyone can design a workout that will kick an athlete's butt or devise an exercise that really burns, but where does that fit? Keep the big picture in mind. Who are you working with? What is their training age? What is their lifestyle? Are they full-time students or professional athletes? Training is more than a method or program; it is a total commitment to personal excellence. Being an effective coach is not about searching for secrets, because there are none. It is about keeping an open mind, continual learning and innovation. Follow the functional path.

Peter Weyand Visit

I was able to meet with Dr. Peter Weyand of Rice University. It was really interesting getting to talk to him directly rather than depending on someone else's interpretation of his ideas. After talking to him, it was clear to me that he and Ralph Mann were essentially saying the same thing in regard to the importance of ground contact time. He also clarified his position on running technique modification; his opinion is that it can't be significantly changed. I certainly understand where he is coming from, but I am not sure I agree.

He made a couple of really key points regarding two myths that keep being passed around. First, the undue emphasis on dorsiflexion of the ankle—there is no basis in biomechanics for this. The ankle dorsiflexion occurs because of what happens at ground contact. Personally, this was a vindication because I feel like I was a voice crying out in the dark on this one. The take-home lesson on this one is, forget cueing all the stuff on dorsiflexion. The other point he made was in regard to the idea of pawing. It does not occur; you can't do it, so forget it.

I am looking forward to further dialogue with Dr. Weyand. He is a very gracious individual, willing to share his ideas with coaches. This is the kind of sport scientist we need more of.

Sprint Mechanics

Anyone who is trying to make someone faster knows that ultimately it is about where the rubber meets the road— ground contact. The goal is very simple: Put more force into the ground in a shorter amount of time. I wish it were as simple as dead lifting more weight. Improving maximal strength is one factor, but not the only factor. I do not want to try to oversimplify this, but to make this complicated would also be a mistake.

There is no doubt that getting someone stronger in terms of maximum strength will make one faster, especially at younger training ages, but my experience has shown that you soon reach the point of diminishing returns. More time in the weight room will not result in more improvement; it must be coupled with a sound overall approach. Running mechanics must be trained. They must be trained to take advantage of the body's natural reflexes—the stumble reflex and the cross extensor reflex.

Technique training should not be mechanical and cognitive, rather it should tune into the wisdom of the body to improve body awareness, posture, and efficiency. When I look at the sprint, I look at four zones: starting, acceleration, top speed, and finishing. Each zone has different technical requirements that must be addressed. Supporting those technical factors are various approaches to strength and power development to enhance each of the zones. A major goal of technical training is to link those zones into a seamless whole that rhythmically flows into the unified whole, the 100-meter sprint.

In order to do that, I use a systematic approach that I have evolved over the past 25 years—The PAL Paradigm. (For a detailed explanation see our book *Sport Specific Speed—The 3S System*). PAL is an acronym for posture, arm action and leg action. All technique work is based on this paradigm. Rather than breaking the sprint stride into too many parts, the PAL paradigm focuses on larger movements that are natural and take advantage of the wisdom of the body. Gerard Mach, former National Coach of Canada, has been a big influence on my thinking in the evolution of this system. Most of his drills are *not* technique drills; they are drills to develop specific strength. My interpretation of Bosch and Klomps' drills is the same—that they are not designed as technique drills. Every time you sprint you should be working on technique. Underlying technique is rhythm and relaxation. Everything must be done in a smooth, flowing manner. The key is to work on mechanics without being mechanical.

The comment has been made several times that there is no research to back all of this. Look at the work of Pavo Komi, and the research of Ralph Mann. There is substantial research, both kinetic and kinematic, on sprint mechanics. Just like any science it is also subject to interpretation.

The Obvious

Look for the obvious first. What made me think about this was an incident that happened the other day. The wireless mouse on my laptop was not working. Panic ensued, because without my mouse I have to use the touch pad, which drives me nuts. So instead of looking at the most obvious thing, the surface the mouse was on, I started resetting the mouse, and checking connections. I even changed the battery, but to no avail. It still would not work.

Then I did the most simple and obvious thing. I put a notepad on the glass surface and, lo and behold, it worked. How often do we do similar things in coaching? The moral of this story is that before looking for exotic solutions, look for the obvious. Sometimes the answer is right in front of you. It does not require biomechanical analysis. It just requires simple powers of observation and common sense.

More Thoughts on Running Mechanics and Technique Training

Strength and force application are a big factor, but not the only factor. Sure, everything is centered on optimizing ground contact, but you must address technique. The question is, how?

Pawing drills are not technique drills. You do not paw when you sprint; that is one example. Getting too far away from actual sprinting with too many segmented drills does not help technique. The drills may indirectly help technique by strengthening through larger ranges of motion. In fact, if you really study Gerard Mach's writing, his drills are not technique drills. They are for power endurance or specific strengthening. For example, the "B" series of pawing-type drills are for functional hamstring strengthening, not technique.

We also need to differentiate technique during different zones of the sprint. Starting and acceleration demand different drills and different training emphasis than does top speed. There is so much bad information out there that creates confusion. I think we need to go back to the basic action of sprinting, thoroughly understand that and compare our sprinters to what we know of proper mechanics. Then derive a plan to improve that individual. Remember, technique also changes with regard to level of development. How you work on technique is important. Without a good foundation of strength it is difficult to achieve sound sprint mechanics. The argument then becomes, how do you work on strength? A hint: It is more than a dead lift and it is more than weights. There is a lot of remedial work!

Athletic Darwinism: Last Man or Woman Standing

Since last year I have been following the results of the teams and individuals from the NCAA Division I Cross Country championships. Many people have bemoaned the fact that we cannot produce distance runners in this country. In my opinion, you need look no farther than the NCAA Cross Country meet. Cross country has taken on a life of its own, with a rankings and a point system to help earn large berths to nationals. This forces teams to compete more than they should, which eventually takes its toll. That toll is taken during outdoor track season. It will be interesting to see how many of the top 25 male and female runners are running effectively by outdoor nationals in track, or even running at all.

I know as a collegiate coach, cross country was a step in preparation for outdoor track. Fortunately, we were not forced to run indoors, which helped put the focus on results where they counted—outdoor track. With the focus on continual performance, development takes a back seat. Only the naturally strong and gifted will survive. Survive not thrive, is that what we want?

Anson Dorrance

Last night, I finished reading *The Man Watching*, by Tim Crothers, a biography of Anson Dorrance, women's soccer coach at the University of North Carolina. It was an interesting read on many levels. I have been a close observer of Anson for years.

Certainly you have to admire his success in terms of winning numerous NCAA championships and a 94-percent winning percentage in all games played. Anson certainly has his detractors, which the book addresses; I am not one of them. We all have our faults and he readily admits his.

I had the opportunity to work with his team in the spring of 1997 and then again in the winter of 1999. It was great to see the system in operation. He is always looking for an edge, which is one example of what it takes to be great. UNC is not for every girl; there is an emphasis on toughness and competitiveness that runs contrary to the accepted role of women in society. He works hard to encourage competition and physical and mental toughness through his famous "competitive cauldron."

Everything in practice is recorded, an idea he picked up from Dean Smith. The players know where they stand at all times in the ranking system he has devised. This is a system that works for Anson at UNC with his assistants and his personality. If I have one criticism, which in many ways is also a compliment, it is that the players who played for him try too hard to institute the UNC system in total at their schools. There is only one UNC and one Anson Dorrance. He has the ability to get players to fit his system—that is crucial—and he always has great depth that other schools cannot match. He can get girls who are willing to walk on and sit for three or four years to wait their turn to play. This does not happen at other places. The women who sit at other places quickly become malcontents or quit.

My other personal experience was getting to see the recruiting process from a personal perspective. My daughter was recruited by UNC, clearly as a walk-on, but one of the 50 girls each year who receive recruiting letters. It was amazing to read those letters, as he is a great communicator. He was very gracious in recommending my daughter to one of his former players who is the coach at Rice University. It was the right school for her, but I know the experience of the UNC Soccer Camp and the interaction with Anson was very special to my daughter. I know as parents, my wife and I appreciated his candor and honesty with our daughter. If you are interested in excellence you need to read this book.

The following quote sums up what he is about and his approach:

> *I saw that my strength in coaching is having the courage to constantly deal with the athletes that unconsciously try to take things a bit easier, and the way I'd lose the respect of my team is not by being demanding enough, not making a passionate, stressful investment. My challenge would be to never surrender my standards to be more popular with my team, but to push my players to transcend ordinary effort in every training session and every match.*

Experience

The book *Mavericks at Work: Why the Most Original Minds in Business Win*, by William C. Taylor and Polly G. Labarre, really got me thinking about experience. I value and trust my experience, but I also realize that it can be a restraining factor. It is not so much about experience; it is really what you do with your experience that counts. I know that sometimes experience results in an approach that is too judgmental; it restrains me and does not allow me to keep an open mind. It is too easy to be trapped into being limited by your experience.

Somewhere in *Mavericks at Work*, an executive they were interviewing said that to be successful and keep progressing he needed to start out each day stupid. Start each day with a clean slate, look at the familiar as unfamiliar, keep learning, stay open to new ideas, re-evaluate old ones as there may be something there that you missed. Look forward without losing perspective on the past, but above all, stay in the moment. Seek out differing and even opposing ideas. (I know this is hard for me, but it is something I need to work on.) Study them for their merit, not their faults.

This is all part of the functional path approach. It is not a one-way street, but a busy street with many intersections that pass through many diverse neighborhoods. Don't get caught in the no-turn lane, because if you do, you might miss a new and exciting discovery.

Another Innovative Idea: Chocolate Milk!

Dr. Joel Stagger at Indiana University actually researched this idea. He stumbled upon it because he is also a swim coach. He was looking for something practical and inexpensive that he could give his swimmers after morning workouts to ensure they were replenished. He came up with chocolate milk because it has all the correct nutrients to speed recovery. Before you judge this, remember 35 years ago they were still telling us to limit water consumption because it would make us sick during exercise!

Results as a Validation?

There is not a more results-oriented person than me. However, as I have stated previously, when I judge a system of athletic performance, my criteria is to look at what someone does with what they have. If you have a bunch of sprinters who have 11.00 ability and eventually you get them to run consistently 11.00, then you have succeeded.

The following comment regarding Frans Bosch struck a tender nerve with me: "In the Netherlands his ideas are supported, but did this really influence the performance level in the Netherlands?" This is the kind of thinking that really sets me off. I am not sure whether or not he is working with the best sprinters in the Netherlands. So how is he doing with those that he is working with? If it were just about results then we should all defer to Trevor Graham; he certainly produced results, but what happens when you take away the medicinal aids and factor in the times that most people ran before they came to him? I know from personal experience that I was no different as a combined event coach when I was coaching decathletes who were scoring in the mid 6,000-point range than later when I had decathletes score in the 7,900s.

All of sudden, people were more interested in what I had to say. That always bothers me. Let's get real, judge someone by what they do with what they have. I have the utmost respect for some of the anonymous high school coaches who, year after year, produce consistently fast performers at their level. Who knows about Patrick McHugh at North Shore Country Day School in Winnetka, Illinois, who produced a state-caliber sprinter without a track? That is how you judge coaching. Remember, talent + coaching = champions.

Our job is to help the people we work with be the best they can be, to reach their potential. Not everyone can be a medal winner, but everyone can take satisfaction in the race they run.

Words

Words are important. Words are a key aspect of communication— both verbal and written. I was taught a long time ago in a teaching methods class at UCSB that words create images and images create action. Nothing in the intervening years has disproved this concept. As far as I am concerned this is precisely why the field of strength and conditioning is so confusing at the present time. There is no accepted lexicon of training. Everybody is trying to make up terms that have no basis in application, much less science. I do not know about you, but I am confused. Is movement prep warm-up? If it is, then call it warm-up. Is prehab remedial work or an injury prevention routine? If it is, then call it that. Is a matrix a circuit? If it is, then call it that. I have been guilty of this at times and I am working hard to be clear and not add to the confusion. This goes on and on.

Let's take a step back, look at the big picture and try to see where we are going with all of this. Communication is essential; words that are meaningful and accurate in the description they portray are very important.

Russian Secrets

Who has the Russian secret training methods? When will the next poorly translated secret Russian sprint program be published? Folks, there are no secrets, Russian or otherwise. I am sorry if I sound a bit cynical here, but in my earlier coaching days I admit I was completely infatuated with anything that the Russians did in training. The more I studied, the more questions I had. Then, the more people I met and the more I began to cross reference translations and find people who had seen the methodology first hand, the more I began to doubt.

In the late '80s there were several tours to Russia, or more precisely, the Soviet Union, where American coaches who paid (in dollars, not rubles), could go to study the Russian methods. I never went but I know many who did. I really doubt if they saw the real deal. They were fed the KGB misinformation that we were reading in the '70s, but they swallowed it hook, line and sinker. They showed them what they wanted to show and told them what they wanted to hear. Now there are some new books available by Russian training experts. I have gotten several e-mails asking if have read them. I have not, but in many ways I have. Looking at a summary and the table of contents, it is the same recycled KGB misinformation that I was reading in the 1970s.

Stress to Stress

Carl Valle said something to me in an e-mail that struck a resonating cord. Can you be too specific? Is it possible to increase pattern overload from too many highly specific movements in training? I think you can. Training for an activity is just that, training to prepare to do that activity. It is not the activity itself. The most specific movement is the activity itself. Each repetitive activity brings with it the potential for a certain pattern overload. That is inherent in the activity.

In the search for specificity of training we may actually be adding to that overload. My basic mantra for a long time has been, train to play. Understand the demands of the activity and prepare the body to tolerate those demands by progressive overload of sport-appropriate movements that do not add stress to stress. I really do not think that a pitcher will forget how to pitch if every movement in training is not highly specific. In fact, I know that executing general movements that work both sides of the body will significantly enhance pitching performance and reduce injuries.

I have never worked with golf, but I find it very interesting studying golf conditioning programs. It is difficult to see where golf coaching ends and conditioning begins. Basic rational movements and weight transfer activities will significantly improve the golf swing without imitating the golf swing. If you want to improve the golf swing and understand the movements of the golf swing, then train movements that enhance the quality of the recruitment of those muscles that stabilize, reduce and produce force.

General and transitional (special) strength should lead to specific strength. Specific strength is resistance or assistance that seeks to imitate the movements of the sport or skill. This should only occupy a small portion of the actual training time. For the past four years I have worked closely with Jim Richardson, the coach of the University of Michigan women's swim team to design their dry land training program. Very little of the program is trying to imitate the swim strokes on dry land, as it is virtually impossible to do. They groove those strokes in the water with thousands of repetitions. The purpose of the dry land program is to work on strengthening movements that will enable them to get in better positions in the water. If you saw the dry land program you probably would not immediately recognize it as a dry land training program. The movements are sport appropriate, so they get the swimmers strong to enhance their work in the water. In summary, think sport appropriate, not sport specific.

Talk the Talk and Walk the Walk

Many talk the talk but very few actually walk the walk. Words are cheap and easy. Anyone can talk about commitment and excellence; that is easy because it does not actually take commitment or excellence. It is not about signs on the wall, or slogans on a t-shirt, it is about actions. Walk the walk—actions speak louder than words. Be consistent. Demand intensity, concentration and effort from yourself daily, and the athletes you work with will follow. Do not settle for anything less.

To be remarkable demands a remarkable approach. No excuses. I have heard them all. Adversity is opportunity. If you don't have enough time, then emphasize intensity. If you do not have enough equipment, then improvise. If you don't have space, then reorganize your workouts. Being remarkable means getting it done. A champion is a champion every day, not just on game day. A champion works when no one else is around to see what they are doing. A champion does not talk, they do—they walk the walk. I recently saw an interview with Pete Carroll; he gets it. He sets the tempo as a coach. He preaches to his players, "You can't choose when you go hard," so he sets the tempo by being totally involved, and he demands the same from his assistant coaches. Because they do it, the players do it. He walks the walk.

Hamstring Pulls Guaranteed: Magic Six-Week Program

If you want to pull hamstrings then spend a lot of time focused on training the hamstring muscles in isolation. Do hamstring curls at least twice a week and try to fit in another day if possible. Be sure to go as heavy as you can and really emphasize the eccentric phase by slowing down the lowering action. If you do not have one, go out and buy a $400 ham/glute machine and add that into the program. That really gets a burn once you master the technique. When you are out on the field as part of warm-up, be sure to throw in a couple of sets of the secret Russian Hamstring curls; you really get a burn on that one. Oh yes, I almost forgot, be sure to do at least ten minutes of static stretching on the hamstrings before you do anything, because everybody knows that stretching prevents hamstring pulls.

Another key aspect of the hamstring pull program, is to do as much running on a high-speed treadmill as possible, that will reinforce over-striding which in combination with everything else will get those hamstrings pulled. I know with this program you will have close to 100-percent success pulling hamstrings; just look at Major League Baseball and the NFL—it works.

The State of Coaching

One night on C-SPAN, I was watching a program broadcast from the Cato Institute on the state of the U.S. Military, focusing on leadership. The first speaker highlighted some of the failings of U.S. military commanders. Three items that he mentioned made me think immediately about coaching. They were: 1) Ahistorical, 2) Technologically infatuated, and 3) Culturally clueless.

Let's look at these in the context of coaching:

Ahistorical: Most coaches who I talk to today have no historical context. They think that everything is new, invented by some guru. I strongly believe that in order to know where you are going you have to know where you have been. There is very little that is new. For example, vibration training is not new, it has been used for at least 30 years. Where did it come from? How was it used? Those are things we must know to make better use of it as a training method today. Understanding historical context always means that we will learn from others' mistakes. Remember, those who ignore history are condemned to repeat it.

Technologically infatuated: We have a fascination with technology, with machines that go beep. The more dials, lights and cables the better. Wrong! Coaching is about teaching the athlete to be better in tune with their bodies. It is not about bigger and better machines. The body is a very high tech machine. We are, as Kelvin Giles says, "performance engineers." Coaching is high touch not high tech.

Culturally clueless: Do we really understand the culture that we are working in? The athlete today at every level has so much more going on (good and bad) in their lives, than when I first started coaching 37 years ago. I would love to turn back the clock on some things, but it is not going to happen. Our culture of affluence and instant results is the culture we must work in. That does not mean that you should compromise your principles, but it does mean being more aware. It does mean being a better communicator.

Context, Context, Context

A reader sent me the following e-mail:

I have a question regarding your thoughts on the Vertimax for training female athletes, ages 14-18 years old. Next, it appears most of your Olympic lifting is performed with dumbbells. Is there any particular reason for the method? Are you against barbell exercises for those lifts?

I really try to stay away from evaluating products or equipment so I will keep my comments very general. The Vertimax is a good tool, but for the money, especially with that age of athlete, there is so much more that needs to be done to improve jumping. In short, look at the context of the people you are training; first teach them good jumping and landing mechanics. Then take them through a systematic plyometric progression where the emphasis is on quality and intensity, not volume. Then, if you think you still need it, go to technology.

I am not against Olympic lifting with a bar, but my basic reason is quite simple. In many situations I work with there is not enough time to spend four-to-six weeks teaching technique with the bar. I must get them training. The dumbbell will accommodate to the person, the bar will not. I can achieve really good pulling technique within one or two sessions and then be on my way training and producing results. Once again, look at the context. If I were working with heavy throwers or American football, then in order to achieve sufficient overload relative to their mass, I would use a bar. In other sports, especially sports like basketball where body proportions mitigate against using a bar, I can achieve the desired results with dumbbells. You can go heavy with dumbbells! Also, remember the reason why you are using Olympic lifts is to develop explosive power. Olympic lifts with dumbbells, kettlebells and sandbags allow me to achieve maximum power production by releasing the implement.

Mile Run Tests

I do not believe in mile run, two-mile run or Cooper tests as fitness tests for intermittent sprint or transition game athletes. First, they send a message that to be successful in these sports is only about endurance. Training for endurance, which they have to do to run well on any of these tests, makes you slow. The last things I want to see are slow basketball or soccer players. Endurance is only one part of the equation.

I would prefer a Beep test to test fitness. Bangsbo's Yo-Yo Intermittent Recovery test is a good test. It is an incremental stage test of twenty-meter shuttle runs with a five-second break between each shuttle. This gives you a starting point to see where the player is in terms of fitness. It is a test that can be incorporated throughout the season. My philosophy of fitness testing is to not use it to disqualify someone, but to determine where they are and develop a program that will get their fitness to a high level in the context of the demands of the game they are playing. In my book, *Athletic Development,* there is extensive treatment of this concept.

Also, with a team, I am more interested in how the team performs than the individuals. I will determine a team average and standard deviations from the mean results and then set team goals for improvement. It is the team that wins or loses, not an individual. For some reason this is a hard concept for coaches to accept, but it works. Remember also that the order of training is to get strong, get fast and then get fit. When you do it that way getting fit is much easier. Oh yes, don't forget to play the game! That will do wonders to get you fit for the game.

Failure

Have you ever failed? I was asked this by someone recently. It seems like a superficial question until you think about it a bit. Sure, I have failed and I hope that I will continue to fail at times. The key is that you learn from your failures and your mistakes. I am convinced that if you are not trying new things and pushing the envelope then you are not getting better. When you do that, failures and setbacks will occur. If you stay in your comfort zone and never take risks, you will not progress.

Failure can be very painful and uncomfortable but if you have sound core beliefs and a good support system then failure will only be an obstacle to overcome. I firmly believe that adversity creates opportunity. Much of the effect of adversity is how you react to it. If you let it defeat you then it will. Success can be blinding; it can allow us to delude ourselves into thinking we are better than we are. Ultimately, it is about putting failure and success into context and keeping perspective.

I have had experiences with two major programs that in many ways were failures. The net effect of those two experiences was to grow and develop, to sharpen my core beliefs, to find out who my friends were and to pick up and move forward. The goal is to move onward and upward!

Excellence

One of my mottos has always been: training the best to be better. It is not easy to be the best and to want to get better, and then actually do it. It is easier to be average. I hear all the excuses. It is not easy to be excellent. You have to keep working, sometimes when you don't want to and no one is around. You have to keep learning. When you think you know it all, you are done.

Right now, after my trip to Holland, I am reading a book about Charlie Weis (former Notre Dame football coach), reading another book about Steve Wozniak (one of the founders of Apple Computer, Inc.), and starting to get more into working with rugby. I am fired up about coaching and being the best I can be. We must have high standards to expect the athletes to perform. We must set high demands for ourselves as coaches. I would like to challenge all of you to strive to be the best. What have you done today to improve yourself? What have you done today to improve your athletes, both as people and as athletes?

Training Information

***Sports Illustrated* now has a regular feature highlighting an athlete's training.** I think this is an interesting idea but it does not quite go far enough. It appears that they are looking for the unusual and out of the ordinary. There is no good attempt to explain the exercises with any depth (I certainly understand that *SI* is not a training journal, but an entertainment magazine). However, with the paucity of information they present, the potential to confuse people is great. Coaches and athletes are very impressionable and often will blindly copy things they see in a magazine without any analysis. The positive side is that it exposes people to the idea that training is necessary to prepare to play.

It can be misleading to provide misinformation because it is often a snapshot of the training taken out of context. For example, in one issue a high school conditioning coach presents three of his key exercises. One of the exercises is sprints using the parachute for resistance. One of the key coaching points he emphasizes on this drill is keeping the arms at a 90-degree angle throughout the sprint. That is perpetuating an old idea about arm action. In fact, the arm angles in sprinting are quite dynamic. In front, the angle closes to less than 45 and on the back to around 110 degrees. Keeping the angle at 90 degrees is inefficient and causes the athlete to sprint with undue tension.

Exercise Comments: The Box Squat

One week, I posted a picture of the Dutch BMX cycling team doing box squats. I was asked at that time to comment on the exercise. This is my opinion based on my experience and research where available.

I assume the rationale for using the box squat with this group of athletes was to work on basic strength in the acceleration phase of the start. The BMX rider must go from a dead stop up to top speed in a very short period of time. There is fairly high resistance during this time, hence the assumption that this would be more concentric-strength dominant.

All of that being said, I would not use the box squat for this. I think traditional squatting starting with body weight moving across a spectrum to heavy external resistance would be more appropriate. When they could handle five to six sets of four reps with a relatively heavy load then I would introduce six-second isometric hold squats (holding at bottom position) and exploding out. Following that, I would progress to squat jump with no counter movement with about 50 percent of body weight for three to four sets of six. The last step in the progression would be deloading squats with a heavy sandbag. Sandbag on the lowering and drop off on the jump.

Personally, I have never used box squats because I have always felt that there are better ways to accomplish the same objective. In my opinion, the loading on the spine when on the box is not worth the risk. I know this is a very popular exercise in certain schools of training, but I think there are better ways to achieve starting strength.

Observations and Ideas Stimulated by the Coaches' Platform Conference in Holland

These are not necessarily original ideas, but my experience in Holland stimulated me to reflect on these.

It is what you do with what you have. Holland is a nation of around 14 million people. They do more with what they have than many other, much larger, countries. It is really about optimizing and directing your resources.

Coaching is the key. Facilities are nice, but human resources trump facilities.

Good coaching demands a blend of art and science. Coaches must have an eye and a feel for movement. You do not learn that in the lab or the classroom, you learn it through practice. To a certain extent you have it or you don't, but it can be improved.

Innovation and change are not always comfortable or popular. Innovators can be even less popular.

The ability to see the same problem with different eyes is essential for progress.

Monitoring training is essential. Now the challenge is to agree on what is meaningful to monitor.

Inactivity and decline of fitness is not just a U.S. problem.

Good coaches are generalists who have a broad base of preparation that allows them to see the big picture.

Early specialization causes more problems than it solves.

Management of the extended competitive season is one of the biggest problems in sports today.

Coaching: The Management Function

Coaching is so much more than writing a workout. I was reminded of this again recently, when I started working with the Sarasota Exiles Rugby Club. Without managing the workout properly a great workout can quickly turn into chaos. There are three realms of coaching management:

1. Training Session Management—This means managing the structure and implementation of each and every training session. I know personally, I spend up to 40 minutes before certain workouts setting up and making sure all equipment is working, and that everything is where it needs to be. All personnel need to clearly know their responsibilities. Everyone must have a copy of the workout with everything detailed as to time segments, responsibilities, etc.

2. Injury Management—As athletic development coaches we must learn to help athletes at all levels manage their injuries. Most injuries in prolonged seasons or contact sports are of the nagging variety that must be planned around in the training. Our job, along with the physical therapist and ATC, is to keep the player fit to play and not make the injury worse. It sounds harsh, but that is the reality of big time sport.

3. Competition Management—Folks, this is where the rubber meets the road. Precompetition warm-up should be orchestrated like a fine symphony. In competition, warm-up and attention to player needs is essential. I am appalled that in the NFL, the strength coach is often used as the *get-back* coach to keep players away from the sidelines. That is demeaning and has no place in the profession. There has to be more to do during the game than that.

Also, in competition, work individual routines in regards to hydration and nutrition. Be sure to have a warm-up again before the second half or a break in play. For example, when Steve Odgers was Director of Conditioning for the White Sox, all bench players went into the locker room after the sixth inning and warmed up in anticipation that they might pinch run, pinch hit or be a late-inning replacement. This also goes a long way toward preventing injury.

All three management realms will go a long way toward determining your effectiveness as an athletic development coach.

The Words "Matrix" and "Spectrum"

As coaches we tend to use words that take on a life of their own. I know I over-use the words spectrum and spectrum training. Another word that I am getting a lot of questions on is matrix. When everything is a matrix, then what is a matrix?

Remember, words create images and images create action. In my mind, I have a very well-defined use for the word matrix in my system; it is a particular dumbbell routine that Gary Gray and I developed in 1996. It simply consists of three different exercises, done in all three planes for three repetitions, repeated three times. To me it is nothing more than that.

As far as spectrum goes, I define spectrum as a broad range of related values, qualities, ideas or activities. Each physical quality that we train is trained across a spectrum. For example, with the strength-training spectrum, according to Vladimir Zatsiorsky, "Exercising at varying levels of resistance causes differences in metabolic reactions, intramuscular coordination, and biomechanical variables and intermuscular coordination." The goal here is not to criticize anyone or say that my ideas are right and someone else is wrong; rather, it is to simplify and be exact in terminology to facilitate communication, and make teaching and learning easier.

The Medici Effect

I am just finishing reading *The Medici Effect* by Frans Johansson, for the second time. I have this habit of reading really high impact stuff a second time to cull even more detail. This is not about the Italian Renaissance, it is about ideas, creativity and innovation.

The basic contention of the book is that breakthrough ideas occur at the intersection of ideas, concepts and cultures. I guess we are always looking for verification or affirmation, but this is certainly the approach I have used throughout my career. I have learned and adapted across sports and disciplines. For example, many of my current ideas on planning come from business planning and forecasting. In order to be the best it is imperative to look across disciplines and even cultures. It is too easy to get locked into one approach or one method and become very narrow. This does not challenge you or your athletes. Too many people become limited by their knowledge. Our current knowledge should only serve as a starting point, not an anchor holding us back.

I know throughout the years, when I thought I already knew something I was setting myself up for failure. The author feels that broad education and self-education are two keys to learning things differently. Johansson says,

"We must employ tactics that allow us to learn as many things as possible without getting stuck in a particular way of thinking about those things." Assimilating and applying the ideas presented in this book will definitely allow you to see things missed by others. I really think this is what Frans Bosch and Ronald Klomp have done in their book, *Running: Biomechanics and Exercise Physiology in Practice*. They have gone beyond the traditional approach to coaching running and speed development. They have looked outside the field and viewed the body with different eyes. The work of Bosch and Klomp epitomizes the Medici Effect.

Real Functional Training

I received this e-mail from a friend of mine. It speaks volumes about things that used to be done, why we have the problems we have today, and what we need to do better.

> I spent most of the afternoon with my 70-year-old father-in-law bailing, stacking and putting up the last cutting of hay from his fields. We stood on a wagon that swayed and shifted as it was pulled around the bumpy field by the tractor while we lifted, carried and stacked the 40-80-pound bales of hay, while the tractor and wagon were in motion. We then unloaded 200 bales and stacked it in a barn. This involved carrying those same bales while walking across bales you have already stacked. Obviously, modern technology in the form of tractors, hay balers and elevators make the job easier, but it occurred to me that the balance, power and strength endurance necessary to complete this task is considerable, and my 70-year-old father-in-law who weighs all of 145 pounds was right in the middle of it with me. As he puts it, he doesn't work as fast as he used to, but he can still get the job done. At a time in life where I begin worrying about my patients falling and breaking a hip, he's riding a wagon and carrying bales of hay. If a sailor has "sea legs," my father-in-law has "farmers' legs." I look at the things I do with the patients I see and the folks I train and much of it is based on development of some of those same qualities.

So much of what we do in training and rehab is done in a very sterile and controlled environment. We are failing our athletes and patients with this approach. The real world is alive, challenging, proprioceptively demanding and chaotic. That is how we need to prepare.

Answers to Various Questions

What do you recommend for recovery *between sets of working with say, a basketball or soccer player for sprinting?*

I recommend proper program design and practice organization. If it is speed work, do longer lines for longer rest. Carefully sequence activities leading into and out of the speed work. Follow speed work with a drill that emphasizes speed of movement and thought in a tactical situation.

This rest debate brings to my mind another subject, the Barry Ross method of training his sprinters. Vern, if you are familiar with it, would you mind commenting?

Someone sent me the book about a year ago (*Underground Secrets to Faster Running*). I read it, but did not find anything revolutionary in it. Perhaps I missed something. Maybe I should go back and read it again. What do you think?

A colleague asked me to comment on my statement, "I have a system that I have evolved over the years. It works for me, in the situations where I am able to apply it hands on." My reply:

As you know having worked with you and your staff for a year-long consultation, there are things that I can do that are not repeatable. It is the sum of my experiences. That does not mean that a system cannot be repeated; it should be repeatable or it is not a system. The mistake people make is to copy everything. I know that you have taken aspects of the system I introduced and added your personal experience and knowledge to make it better for North Shore Country Day school.

What would be the ideal curriculum to prepare someone for an entry-level athletic development/strength and conditioning job, besides the usual anatomy and biomechanics? Maybe this is something your book will address, but I would like to know what you think the young professional needs to know upon leaving college.

This is a very good question. First of all, get extensive hands-on, practical experience under direct supervision of a trained professional in an athletic setting, not a Gold's Gym or a health club. There should be extensive course work in applied biomechanics as well as several courses on training theory including training plan projects. Each student should have to produce a training video or an instructional package on an area of their choice. They must take what in the old days we used to call "activity classes", where they have to show fundamental proficiency to be able to demonstrate movements. Go long on practice supported by theory.

More Random Thoughts on Recovery

The key to recovery and proper adaptation is good planning.
Plan the recovery days. It goes back to Bill Bowerman's hard/easy principle: An easy session following a hard session to allow recovery. Good planning will take care of a high percentage of the problems. Plan 14-day microcycles instead of seven, to allow for better distribution of work and recovery.

The ability to recover from the training and adapt is the essence of the whole process. My experience has taught me that this is highly individual. To address this individuality in adaptive response to training I use the term recoverability. That is the subjective assessment of the athlete's ability to recover from the stress of training. Assessing recoverability is very subjective—it demands a day-to-day, session-to-session coaching presence to constantly assess and evaluate the athlete's recoverability. Remember, there are fast adapters and slow adapters, and everyone does not progress at the same rate.

External means of recovery like massage, sauna, contrast baths and laser therapy can all add stress if overused. These external means, if used indiscriminately, will short-circuit the adaptive process. A few years ago, one of the NFL teams was having their players get a massage everyday postworkout in the off-season. To me, that is overkill.

Also, more recovery modalities, treatments and therapies cannot make up for bad training design. Recovery methods should not be used to enable even more and harder work.

As I said the other day, I strongly believe that during certain periods of training the body's natural inflammatory response should be allowed to trigger the adaptive response. I emphasize, *only at certain stages*. I have also tried to only use external methods later in a microcycle, or later in a block when fatigue accumulates, and in essence when the body's own ability to respond needs help. It's not really scientific but highly intuitive.

You have to consider efficiency. If you are working one-on-one with an athlete then a lot of this is practical. In large team settings it is not cost and time efficient. Teaching the athletes how to stretch properly postworkout can help a lot. Large amplitude movements in a swimming pool can aid recovery at little cost.

One aspect of recovery that is seldom addressed is what the athlete does intra-workout. What is done between sprints, between sets to possibly enhance the quality of the next drill or exercise? This should be explored. Carefully look at work-to-rest ratios. This requires very detailed planning that carefully considers each individual's variability. This is also about recoverability.

Last, but not least, carefully consider the demands of the sport. I divide sports into three categories that heavily influence planning of recovery. Impact sports are subdivided into repetitive/chronic lower repetitive impact sports, like distance running; and acute high impact sports, like triple jump and gymnastic landings. Then there are contact sports, like soccer and basketball and lastly collision sports, like American football, rugby, and hockey where there is actual external trauma to the muscle, which demands a whole different approach. Recovery strategies must be developed that are appropriate to each of those situations.

Finally, I would like to recommend an article by Dr. Owen Anderson in *Running Research News*, Volume 21, #6, August 2005, titled, "The Six Step

Recovery Process." It is a very good article that cites relevant research and recommends some practical recovery strategies.

Labels

Eastside, Westside, all about the town. Does it really matter if you are a Westside guy, unless you are in a gang? I despise labels. I guess that does not leave too much wiggle room. A couple of people said the Westside Barbell guys were upset with my post on recovery. I am sure many people were because I had the audacity to question conventional wisdom. Frankly, to be good at what you do, you cannot afford to worship at the altar of a method or hang your hat on one person's ideas. To be the best demands an eclectic approach.

I learned this a long time ago from Bill Bowerman. He proudly acknowledged all the influences that were the ingredients of the Oregon Program. I am all about training. I have a system that I have evolved over the years. It works for me, in the situations where I am able to apply it hands-on. Certain other people have been able to adapt aspects of my system to their situations and create their own systems, and more power to them. To train, you can't just lift heavy, and you can't just sprint; you do what you have to do depending on the demands of the sport and level of development of the athlete. That demands attention to all components of training at all times in different proportions. To define a profession and move forward in training, let's get past all the arguing.

Kelvin Giles on Recovery

Kelvin is with player development for the Australia Rugby Union. He is a coach with vast experience and I certainly attach great value to his comments.

The research and application of recovery modalities in the current age is to be commended as it allows us the opportunity to question our assumptions on the subject. The problem arises when the coach simply jumps on a new fad or idea without any thought. Without any thought we will have a garage full of ice-baths, special drinks, special meals, electrical gadgets and other things that make us glow in the dark.

The key is to understand fatigue and to understand this with reference to the individual. Fatigue is a side effect of training and should not be viewed as some catastrophe. We know that sensible training with suitable recovery can lead to super-compensation. The important word is 'suitable'. On one hand, you could say that for a certain level of fatigue a good night's sleep will be the perfect solution. On the other, you may have to react to the specific fatigue encountered and respond appropriately. Is the fatigue chronic due to a poorly managed program or is it a manifestation of other variables in the athlete's life. Is the fatigue physical, emotional, social or a combination of them all?

I know that I have seen some distinct improvements in recovery from high impact games by the use of ice-baths. The micro-traumas of contact can be more quickly assisted to recovery using this modality. I have seen some workloads improved when, during very hot training conditions, intra-set cold water immersion has helped the athlete. This does not mean that everyone should run out and copy this. These were highly trained athletes in a very controlled environment and the evidence is subjective. The decision was based upon the environment in front of me—I reacted to the stress involved in the session. As stated before, recovery from other sessions was simply a good night's sleep.

If I put my "'grumpy old man" hat" on I would also say that I don't want to get to the position where we spend all our time in recovery and less and less time in pushing out the edge of the envelope. Smart training will still see the athlete taken to their physiological, psychological and structural limits. Too often I have seen individual athletes and teams tapering from a taper where they have entered into a sphere of protection from physical adversity. Recovery must be part of the written program whether one manages it in the intrarep/set/microcycle/phase environment, but you had better have been working hard in-between.

Rethinking Recovery

After you finish working/training the rest should be easy, or is it? There is certainly an increased awareness of the role that recovery plays in training. After all, it is during the recovery and rest period that the adaptation to training takes place. That is precisely why I think we need to rethink some things that are going on now in terms of the application of recovery modalities and therapies. We need to think about what we are trying to achieve with hot/cold contrast baths, ice baths, massage, etc.

What I see happening now with recovery is the same mistake I have seen made in training. If we throw enough stuff at the body it will get better. More is not better in training or recovery. The goal of training is to stimulate adaptation to the training stimulus. Different training stimuli adapt at different rates. The body has a natural healing response to injury and to training, the first phase of which is inflammation. I wonder if, with some of the indiscriminate application of recovery modalities, we are not inhibiting the natural inflammatory response, which triggers the body's natural recovery cascade. I have no research to back this up, just my gut feeling and experience, but it is something we really need to look at. For example, during a general block of training where there is no competition and the amount of technical and tactical work is low, would it be better to leave the body alone and let it repair itself? Would we get a better adaptative response? Use the modalities later in different phases when the athlete is trying to get an edge.

As you know, I am not one to follow the crowd and this definitely is in opposition to what is being accepted as conventional wisdom.

The Day Sport Changed

In October 2006, the Australian sprinter Peter Norman died of a heart attack, aged 64. Most of you probably have no idea who Peter Norman was; he was a 200-meter sprinter who won the silver medal in the 1968 Olympics. The time that he ran that day, 20.06, is still an Australian record. That is all incidental to what happened on the victory stand, however. The winner, Tommie Smith, and the bronze medalist, John Carlos, both of the USA, used the podium to raise their gloved fists in protest of racial inequities in the U.S. What is not known, is that Norman wore an Olympic Project for Human Rights badge on his shirt in support of Smith and Carlos.

I believe that this protest, symbolic as it was, changed sport. Before this protest, sport was considered in isolation from the rest of society. Everyone knew there were problems but sport was considered an island, if you will, an escape. 1968 was a year of turmoil and protest; Martin Luther king had been assassinated that spring, Robert Kennedy was killed that June, and there were protests in the streets against the war in Vietnam. In Mexico City just before the games, thousands of students had rioted in the streets protesting inequality and injustice in Mexico. Hundreds, perhaps thousands, were killed by police, but the games went on.

The gloved fist protest brought the reality of the outside world into the sports arena. As someone who was just starting in coaching it certainly shook my foundation. It caused me to be more sensitive to the athlete outside of practice and the games and above all to be much more socially conscious of the ills of society. In the spring of 1968, I had seen where Tommie Smith grew up in the Central Valley of California. The Joads in Grapes of Wrath had nothing over what he endured growing up. When I saw those conditions, I could not believe this was the U.S.—it looked more like Soweto or the slums of Calcutta.

I hope that the protest by these three athletes was not in vain. Unfortunately, what I see today in the world reminds me of what I saw as a 21-year old, naïve college senior in 1968. Hopefully, the spirit of Peter Norman and his silent support of Smith and Carlos will awaken in all of us a renewed interest and concern for our fellow man and a spirit of tolerance and love. We can use this protest to remind ourselves of our responsibilities as human beings who are privileged to take part in sport.

Real World Coaching

I once made a comment in my blog about "real world coaching" and someone wanted me to explain what I meant by that. To me, real world coaching is getting down and dirty, working in the field, in the weight room, making a long-term commitment with an athlete or a group of athletes, to see them through a training year or a career. It involves dealing with the *24-hour* athlete not this hour's client. It is very labor intensive and involves an ever changing blend of sport science, coaching and, above all, art and feel for the athlete. It can be no tech or high tech depending on the situation. It is about accountability and results; it is coaching as a way of life. A good coach must be equally as committed as any great athlete. It is more than writing workouts; it is being there during the glory times and during the down times. It is not about fame and fortune; it is about personal satisfaction in a job well done. That is real world coaching.

Dave Brubeck

The other night I caught the tail end of an interview with Dave Brubeck regarding his performance at the Monterey Jazz Festival. I admire creative people, and have always been a fan of Dave Brubeck. It was great to hear him and see that he is still just as vibrant and creative as ever. At Monterey he performed a new work called the "Cannery Row Suite" honoring John Steinbeck. As a jazz fan one of my earliest exposures to the genre was listening to Brubeck. In college I used to play his concert at Carnegie hall by the hour. That album got me through many long nights writing papers; in fact, I still listen to it today. He is now at least 84-years old and he continues to tour and produce. When asked why he kept going at age 80, he replied, "Because I want to be better than last time." (He was starting on a multi-city tour of Europe.) That is what it takes to be great!

Thoughts on the Russian Hamstring Exercise

The rush to adopt the Russian Hamstring as a key ACL prevention exercise has many flaws. As far as I am concerned this is another example of the "doctor-as-God syndrome." Because the Santa Monica Sports Medicine Group's study that showed a supposed reduction in ACL injuries in female youth soccer players was sponsored by a doctor, then of course this must be an okay exercise. FIFA endorses it because the doctor is a team doctor for U.S. Soccer. This, perhaps, is one of the most frustrating things I have seen over the years. Things like this take on a life of their own and no one ever questions them.

When the study was being done involving this exercise and several other questionable practices, I spoke to the person designing the study and my comments fell on deaf ears. In fact, I would not let my daughter participate in the study because I thought several aspects of the program were fundamentally flawed. There is so much more to it than what they looked at, but the conclusion that I came to (as flawed as this exercise is and several other things they did) is if you get them doing something, ACL injures will decline!

This is an e-mail I got from Daniel Cipriani, Ph.D., P.T., a great PT and a professor at San Diego State. I think he explains the shortcomings of the so-called Russian Hamstring exercise quite well from a scientific perspective.

I completely agree with you on the Russian exercise not at all reproducing the normal forces of the hamstrings...the hamstrings are a "hip" muscle much more than they are a "knee" muscle...their moment arm at the hip is greater for producing torque. In addition, the hamstrings are generally injured during the late swing phase of running/walking just prior to foot contact, when the muscle is at its longest position (extended knee, flexed hip)...and also right at heel contact, when it is working, first eccentrically control hip flexion followed by concentric hip extension to propel us forward. Lunges would be a better choice as would be Thera-Band eccentrics, replicating the swing phase of gait (let the band pull the swing).

The argument that the hamstrings are necessary for ACL reconstruction is based on misinterpretation of research related to the role of the hamstrings shear by producing a posterior shear force to the tibia. The problem with this finding is the fact that the hamstrings are only effective at producing this significant posterior shear when the knee is flexed at least 70 degrees from full extension (this aligns the distal tendon attachment at the tibia closer to the horizontal plane)...when the knee is near full extension, the hams are not effective at producing a posterior force—and the ACL is at greatest risk when the knee is at near full extension...not flexion.

College Soccer: In-Season Training

Here is a sample of an in-season program, including my thoughts as to why things are done.

TESTING: As far I am concerned this should not be a major emphasis in the fall. This should be emphasized in the winter/spring with the goal being to identify strengths and weaknesses to better direct the off-season training. I recommend the Yo/Yo (Beep test) with a team goal of 15.6 without the goalkeepers. The 300 Shuttle test—the key here is to reflect game fitness in as little difference between the two runs as possible.

CONDITIONING: When the team reports, set team goals. Determine leaders for each area of conditioning, so they are responsible and have ownership. Rather than have extra sessions for someone who does not test well, have a team session instead. The theme should be a little bit, more often. The conditioning sessions do not have to be long and strenuous, they just need to be consistently applied. Training is cumulative. Conditioning should be part of every practice. No single day is a conditioning day, but different components of fitness are addressed in each practice in a sequence, so they are fresh for the games. My thought is that the season is too short and each game too important to have players going into the games with dead legs. In order to do this we need to put our heads together so that the technical and tactical work correlate with the fitness theme for the day.

Do not underestimate the conditioning value of various small-sided games with defined conditions. The key is to look closely at the intensity of the small-sided game and define the conditions to achieve the fitness as well as the tactical objective. The size of the field, number of touches and the number of players will change the work-to-rest ratios, which impacts the component of fitness you are working on. Also consider putting small segments of fitness, speed and speed endurance drills between soccer-specific drills during practice. That breaks it up and makes it more game like. This is the ideal sequence:

Good warm-up every day. Pool recovery session wherever possible, especially Wednesday and Thursday.

Day One—Aerobic emphasis, 30-60 seconds with 1:1 work-to-rest ratio. Lower intensity with shorter rest. Not high volume. Strength train.
Day Two—Speed development and agility work possibly working into speed endurance. Strength train—core work.
Day Three—Emphasize speed endurance. 8-10 seconds in duration with 30-40 seconds recovery. Strength train.
Day Four—Speed acceleration—short and quick. Agility. Strength train—core work.
Day Five—Good, sharp warm-up. Footwork. Get quick.
Day Six—Game.

This obviously must be adjusted when there are multiple games in a week.

PRESEASON: Plan the recovery days first. This will make it proactive not reactive. Look at specific recovery sessions in a combination of work in, and out, of the pool. Good recovery will allow the players to work at a higher percentage of their capacity at all times. Therefore, the sum total training effect of the preseason will be greater than if they are completely torn down. Also, carefully consider time of day for training.

FOLLOWING THE FUNCTIONAL PATH

STRENGTH TRAINING: This should be done at the field. It would be good to have dumbbells in pairs from 12, 15, 20 and 25 and a couple of pairs of 30s. The majority should be in the 10-25 pound range. Have enough so no one is standing around. Have the athletes work in pairs. If they are not lifting they will be doing core work, so that a 15- or 20-minute workout will involve no standing around. It should be total activity for the whole workout.

Lunges and Squats

I cannot choose between these exercises in a total program. They have slightly different functions depending on the level of athlete and the phase of training. Also, where they are used in rehabilitation must be considered. The most basic leg exercise is the single leg squat. That is really the basis of a sound lower extremity strengthening program. The body weight squat is another foundation exercise and serves as the starting point.

Of equal importance to the body weight squat is the lunge, starting anterior and then working into the frontal and transverse planes. The lunge is a more versatile exercise in terms of being able to work in multiple planes. Like the squat, it is an exercise that is always somewhere in the program. Perhaps the most useful variation of the lunge in terms of strengthening the hamstring group, is the lunge and reach.

Simplicity, Innovation and Change

Simplicity, innovation and change. Wow, that is a mouthful, but in my eyes they are all related. To stay the same we must change—that is where innovation comes in. I know I am always trying to find a better way. Innovation is not just change for the sake of change; it is change with a defined purpose. As I have already stated in this blog, simplicity is the key. Sometimes it is no more than changing the sequence of exercises; other times it takes more. But above all, it is simple. I have just finished reading a simple book on simplicity—only a hundred pages. Absolutely brilliant! It is by John Maeda, a professor at MIT (Massachusetts Institute of Technology). It is called, *The Laws of Simplicity (Simplicity: Design, Technology, Business, Life)*. The whole time I was reading the book I could not help but think of the things that have worked consistently well for me over the years. A sequence of exercises like the leg circuit can spin off into a very complex leg strength development program if you don't initially try to make it more than it is.

Another key point regarding simplicity, is that simplicity does not mean dumbing things down. If anything, it is the opposite. I believe that to make things simple you must have a real clue. If you do not, things will easily become complicated. I also could not help thinking about a piece that I heard on the radio the other morning on a popular style of running that is being promoted as the answer to injury-free running. When I got through listening to it, I was confused so I went to the Web site and read the transcript. I am still confused. They are taking a simple, natural activity like running and making it complicated. Play, run like your life depended on it—that is sprinting. Your foot will land correctly. Play, run like you are stalking a meal for two hours—that gives you the perfect gait to run a marathon. Make it simple. As a former javelin thrower that I used to know said: "Get your center of gravity beyond infinity."

Game Fit

What is game fit? In games that require quick starts and stops that are classified as intermittent sprint or transition game sports, what do you have to do to be game fit? If you believe what you see in testing, then it would be the ability to cover as much ground as possible in a twelve-minute run or the ability to run three miles in a certain time. This is where the problem originates; to be game fit requires the ability to start and stop quickly and repeat quick movements in a climate of fatigue. There is no question that in sports like soccer, rugby, basketball and similar sports, having a good aerobic capacity will help with recovery between intense bouts of exercise. You raise that aerobic capacity not by distance running but by doing intervals at the velocity of VO2 max and the accumulation of all the other training that is taking place. Just because a player runs six or eight miles in the course of the game does not mean that they should run six miles continuously in training.

Look at how they accomplish that distance in a game. A great majority of it is walking or slow jogging. However, it is during the quick bursts and the explosive actions that the games are won or lost. This should be a huge clue. Training slow will make you slow and not necessarily fit to play the game.

Facilities and Equipment

Facilities and equipment should never be the determining factor in program design. I always start with the assumption that I have a bare room, or a field with no equipment. If you start with that assumption then the focus is on the athlete and what they need to do to get better. Too often, if facilities, equipment and even to a certain extent, training methodologies become the first determining factors in a program, then we tend to fit the athlete to the facility, equipment or methodology. It should be the other way around; the program should fit the athlete in order to achieve optimum results.

Don't get me wrong, a good training facility can only enhance the training, but it is not 100-percent necessary. I have seen world champions train in what was no more than a closet. The basis of everything you do is manipulating the three movement constants—the body, gravity, and the ground. They will always be there and they travel well. Look at your environment for tools that you can use. Trees and rocks work well; you can climb trees and throw rocks. When those possibilities are exhausted then start looking at equipment that will enhance the program. For example, before I moved to Florida, hill sprints were always a foundation of my speed and speed endurance development programs. Where we live in Florida there are no hills, so I had to improvise. More sled work and work with vests had to suffice. It is not the same but I had to understand how it differed and account for that in the programs. It works—not as well as hills, but it works.

The bottom line is, we are in a results-oriented business. I must admit I would find it hard today to coach without my medicine balls, dumbbells, hurdles, pulley machine, rings and all the other toys I like to use, but if I had to, I would. Remember, simplicity yields complexity.

Respect

Respect is something that you earn; that is something I was always taught. You do not have to be friends with someone to respect someone. Just like discipline, respect starts with self-respect. If you do not respect yourself how can you respect someone else? This leads me to all the taunting and disrespect that is going on today in sport. The essence of competition is to strive together with the competition in order to raise the level of play, and then the best team or individual will win. They will win not by putting down the competition, but by respecting and honoring their effort. It is not possible to be a champion without a worthy opponent.

The Most Important Person is Not Playing in the Game

Who is the most important person? Not the coach, that is for sure; not the parents—you should not know who they are. If they do their job well, the most important person is invisible: the official. The official at any level of sport can have a profound influence on the outcome of the game. His or her ability to pay attention and stay on task to focus on the game is paramount. They do not get to go to the bench to rest. At the youth sport level the official can teach the players more about the game in the course of one game than the coach can in a week. Learning the rules and playing by the rules significantly improves the quality of play and also prevents injury.

One of the reasons for the high rate of injury in youth soccer and girls basketball is poor officiating. The officials lose control of the game and the players play out of control, increasing their chance of injury. Officials must be game fit to be able to effectively officiate a game. This is one of the biggest deficiencies in sport today. I know Major League Baseball has tried to address this. It is becoming increasingly difficult to get officials because of the disrespect and abuse. So I guess it is hard to expect them to be game fit, but if possible, this should be addressed by officiating associations.

Sport Ready

Despite all our advances in sport science and increased sophistication in training, today's athletes are not as *sport ready* as athletes from past generations. They have not paid their athletic dues or, as Kelvin Giles has said, earned the right to train and compete at higher levels. Sure, they have the talent and that is what carries them. Look at the injuries: pulled hamstrings, strained oblique muscles, pulled groins and calf muscles, and even some of the shoulder injuries and non-contact ACL injuries. These injuries could be prevented or significantly reduced with a sound athletic development program that prepares the athletes athletically to withstand the forces involved in running, jumping and throwing.

Look at Martina Navratilova. She is still competing (and competitive) in her 50s. Why? She has paid her dues by preparing athletically. She came out of a system as a youth that prepared the athletes to play by providing them with a rich repertoire of motor skills upon which to build their specific sport skills. Today, we are trying to identify athletes early and then get them into a specific sport as soon as possible. Expose the young athlete to as wide a range of movement skills as possible and demand competence in those skills before they specialize in specific sports.

I am reading an interesting book now by Thomas E. Ricks called, *Making the Corps*. He follows a platoon of recruits through their training at Parris Island. I am not a military person, but I am fascinated by how the Marines are able to mold their recruits into Marines. What I found particularly interesting, is that before they start actual training for any combat, (the specific kill), they are drilled for weeks in the basics of teamwork and communication. This should be a clue. When lives are at stake, they take care of the basics first.

I sincerely maintain that we are putting a generation of athletic lives at stake because we are not taking care of basics. If we keep following this totally dysfunctional path we will see injuries go off the charts. Sure, we will see great performances, but the cost will be high. For my consulting business I am designing a Sport Readiness module for those who engage my services. It has been the most difficult of all the modules to design because of the context of the society and culture we live in. Red light, green light and tag games are basic; hop scotch is basic ACL prevention. Let's get real and wake up. Give the kids a chance by being *FUNdamental*!

Overhead Exercises and the Shoulder

Overhead exercises are not necessarily bad for the shoulder.
This is almost as big a myth as the knee over the toe. The shoulder is designed to allow the arm to move overhead. But we must focus again on linkage. The arm is one of the last links in the kinetic chain (referencing from the ground up). Instead of worrying about overhead activity we should focus on how the arm gets overhead. To understand that, we need to look down the chain at the core and the hips. To get the arm directly overhead requires an inclination of the trunk to allow the head of the humerus to clear the glenoid fossa.

Simply, instead of eliminating overhead activity, work on how the arm is getting overhead. One of the main jobs of the core is to help position the extremities. When we do strict presses and seated behind-the-neck activities, and combine those activities with a high volume of movements that occur in tennis, baseball and swimming, then we are asking for trouble. Instead, focus on hip mobility, core strength, dumbbell pressing movements standing that allow the trunk to help position the arm. See my video, *Functional Shoulder Exercise*, for numerous exercises that address getting to overhead.

Certification

I have received quite a few inquires regarding certification.
I do not and will not offer a certification. There are already too many certifications now. Another certification will only confuse and muddle an already confused field. I offer a mentorship program that is an in-depth educational experience. It offers a blend of hands-on experience and in-

depth theory. The first GAIN (Gambetta Athletic Improvement Network) Apprentorship program was held in 2008. The program continues as a yearly event.

High Tech or High Touch?

I was sent an article from a newspaper in Sydney, Australia, about the Sydney Swans' visit to the highly secret AC Milan High Tech training center. They were visiting the center because AC Milan has had no soft tissue injuries over the past two years. Is there really a secret here or is it that they have paid attention to basics and made sure the players comply? In nine years with the White Sox minor league system we only had five hamstring pulls and six groin pulls. The secret was a high touch approach: doing basic work everyday and ensuring it was done with intensity, concentration and effort.

Which Exercise?

The answer is simple; it is more than selecting an exercise. It is selecting the correct exercises for the individual player's needs. It is what exercise you do and when you do it. Timing is essential. A good exercise during a general training block may be totally inappropriate during peak competition. This is one of the biggest problems we face today as people begin to understand the importance of multiple plane and multiple joint movement. It is more than an exercise!

Bill Bowerman

I have just finished a terrific book that is a must-read for anyone who wants to be a better coach or leader. The title of the book is *Bowerman and the Men of Oregon*, by Kenny Moore. Bill Bowerman was the longtime track and field coach at the University of Oregon, who is now probably better known as one of the founders of Nike. Bowerman is a person who had a profound effect on my coaching career, so I had a strong connection to the book.

He spoke at the first track and field coaching clinic I ever attended in February 1968, when I was a senior at Fresno State. I was thinking about going into coaching, but was still a bit unsure. After sitting in on Bowerman's talks there was no doubt about what I wanted to do: I wanted to be a coach like him. He was passionate, very outspoken and strongly opinionated. He made complicated things simple and easy to understand. Over the years I tried to attend anytime, anywhere, he was doing a clinic. He did not change his foundational beliefs. He was a great innovator.

His ideas on training the middle distance and distance runner are still very relevant today, even though everybody seems to ignore them. He understood adaptation. He understood that his runners had to do more than run. He was an innovator in shoe design in the 1950s by making special shoes for his runners. He was a generalist in that he coached other events and even coached football as an assistant at the University of Oregon. His mantra was, "Stress, recover, improve, that's all training is." If you want to learn about training and read some great stories, read this book. When I finished I could not help but wonder what Bowerman would think of the state of track and field today. I think I know: He would not be happy and he would do something about it.

Time

This is the opening verse and the refrain from one my favorite songs by the Pozo Seco singers:

Some people run, some people crawl
Some people don't even move at all
Some roads lead forward
Some roads lead back
Some roads are bathed in light
Some wrapped in fearful black

Time, oh, time
Where did you go?
Time, oh, good, good time
Where did you go?

I heard this the other day on the radio and it made think about time. In the context of training and rehab nothing could be truer. Training and the subsequent adaptation to training take time. Time is there, so use it. There are two major mistakes that we all make with time:

1. We try to do too much too soon. Progression is forgotten and we put the athlete on a fast track. This is often a fast track to injury. Make time your friend, not your enemy. Understand that there are fast adapters and slow adapters and that they all cannot train the same.

2. We cram too much into too short a time frame. Think fourteen days instead of seven. I know the earth was created in seven, but athletes are created in fourteen. Along with that, get away from the typical 6:1 training-to-rest ratio, and put the rest where you need it, not where it is convenient. For example, we put a recovery day this week on Wednesday. It was great, and things were very positive during Thursday's and Friday's training sessions.

One of the best axioms that I have heard in regard to using time, is to do a little bit more often.

The Profession and Jobs

Here is an important question from a reader:

Take a look at the NBA. There are teams out there right now looking for a new head strength coach but only offering a $45,000 salary with a prerequisite of a NASM (National Academy of Sport Medicine) certification. If this is as good as it gets (becoming a head strength coach coach at a pro level), then maybe it's not that good. Why? I would love to get Vern's insights in the job opportunity market for those young coaches who want to make a career out of this.

The field is undefined. The fact that they require NASM certification speaks volumes about what is wrong with the field and how undefined it is. If they require NASM certification they don't get it, so it is probably not a job worth having.

You must pay your dues. Start coaching at the high school level. You can make more money there than anywhere, plus you learn the ropes.

That being said, do not work for nothing. One internship is all someone needs to do. Interns are now a source of free labor for many people. Once you work for nothing you will always work for nothing. I know that from personal experience. It has taken me 37 years to figure that out. To me, salary is commensurate with proven, not perceived, ability and accomplishments. If you have three years of experience, then the salary should reflect that.

As far as being under the supervision of the trainer, that is our fault for not defining the profession. When I was Director of Conditioning for the White Sox, I was in charge of the minor league trainers. I hired them and occasionally had to fire them. The end result was a great conditioning program that kept players healthy because the trainer had a vested interest in being part of the process instead of being on the outside pointing fingers. With another team it was the opposite experience: every time I turned around my hands were tied. The results spoke for themselves.

Certification and education are not the same. Young people today are spending way too much time and money acquiring certifications that are essentially meaningless. Get out and get experience. Go for a week and observe a Jim Radcliffe at the University of Oregon or a Chris Doyle at the University of Iowa, and then you will see what it is all about.

One of my goals for the rest of my career is to help to define this field.

Breaking It Down

For a long time, I have lived by the motto that simplicity yields complexity. I am continually amazed by how people try to make things complicated. When you think of the human body and its potential for movement, it is complex enough without trying to make it more complicated. I was watching a golf conditioning guy work the other day and I felt sorry for the golfer. He was making it so complicated that Tiger Woods would not have been able to do it. I believe that we must simplify, not complicate. Think of the essentials of movement and what buttons need to be pushed in order to trigger those movements.

If you take a step back and break movements into some basic patterns, it is very simple to see if the individual is efficient in those patterns. If they are not, it is essential to see why and where they are not, and then to construct a program that enhances those movements.

Use one movement to set up another movement. Use one workout to set up another workout. Think about how to build relationships. Remember strength training is no more than pulling, pushing, squatting and rotating. Speed development is no more that extending, bending, and force application against the ground. Even simpler is that it can all be summarized in the performance paradigm: it is the interplay between force reduction, force production and proprioception to lend quality to the movement.

Too Much, Too Soon

Here are some thoughts regarding arm and shoulder injuries in young pitchers. Nowadays, there is too much, too soon because specialization occurs way too early. Prepuberty, in fact pre-high school, athletes should not be just pitching. Every kid on the team should pitch. There should be a limit on the number of games kids can play. They compete too much and do not train enough. They pitch too much and do not throw enough. They play to train; they do not train to play.

Let me explain those points: There should be a ratio of four to five practices to every game. They do not just get out and throw rocks and other objects. Consequently, they have poor arm strength and throwing mechanics that are not developed naturally. These athletes may have a personal pitching coach, but they need to long toss to build specific strength.

Pitch counts are fine, but that does not go far enough. They should have a pitch count limit and only be allowed to pitch once every seven days. No curveballs or other breaking pitches. Only fastballs and change-ups.

Ultimately, these injuries are the result of early specialization. Again, it's too much, too soon. Let them just play. Adults are way too involved. Kids' sports should be about kids. I think televising youth sports has caused the problem to get worse.

Change

I was reading a new book I picked up at the library called *Fast Company's Greatest Hits—Ten Years of the Most Innovative Ideas In Business.* It essentially is a reprint of the best articles from the last ten years of *Fast Company* magazine. The article that immediately caught my eye was titled "Making Change" by Alan Deutschman, from May 2005. I have always been fascinated by change from both an institutional perspective and an individual perspective. Change is a constant, there is no question about that, but can you really change behavior? As a coach with a messiah complex I have always wanted to believe that you could, but it is difficult. This article underscored how difficult change is. For example, people faced with death from heart problems tend to not change their diets.

So how do we change or even modify behavior? When I have seen change happen, it has taken unbelievable personal commitment and willingness on the part of the person wanting to change. They must want to change. They need support and guidance that is firm and fair. They have to be taken out of their comfort zone. This is not a religious experience; it is blood, sweat and tears. Sometimes it means swallowing your pride. Basically, it requires running a different script for your life.

Turn Back the Clock

Saturday afternoon, I was watching the ESPN nationally televised high school football game between Byrnes High School in South Carolina and Belle Glade High School in South Florida. (Why I was watching a high school football game on a summer Saturday afternoon I do not know.) I was struck with the thought, as I was watching the game, that this was all way over the top. The closer I get to 60, the more I long for the good old days when things were simpler.

A road trip was a three- or four-hour bus ride in a school bus, not a flight across country. A pregame meal was what your mom packed for lunch. In those days you had to wash your own uniform. (One guy did not all season and he was very offensive.) There were no passing leagues in the summer, we just got together and played games. A big coaching staff consisted of three coaches. If you wanted an off-season program you met your friends at the YMCA and lifted weights. (Heavy all the time and squats three times a week.) Ignorance is bliss. The only name on the uniform was that of your school. Corporate sponsorship meant you sold an ad in the game to the local car dealer. A guy who weighed 250 pounds was *huge*! In basketball, a guy like me who was 5'11" could jump center against the big guys who were 6'3" or 6'4". Pitchers threw 300 innings. There were not many pulled hamstrings either because we either did not know what a hamstring was, or we could not run fast enough to pull them. Choosing a shoe was really tough—Chuck Taylor All Stars—high tops or low cut, black or white, and boy, were they expensive: $9.95. The parents were fans; they did not run the teams, the coaches did. Cheerleaders actually cheered. They also wore the jewelry, not the players.

I know these are revolutionary thoughts, but those were the good old days.

Good Coach, Bad Coach

Coaching is my life. I have been a coach for 37 years. I decided I wanted to be a coach when I was still in high school. I was fortunate to have a great high school basketball coach, Mr. Charles Kuehl; he was also a history teacher, which inspired me to also be a history teacher. The older I get, the more I appreciate the lessons and values he taught. He was a stickler for detail and discipline. I know now he taught us life lessons. He kicked me out of practice for seven straight days because I was arguing calls; on the eighth day, I finally shut up. Not a word was said. I was just a little slow to get the lesson. He knew that taking away the game would be more punishment than running laps. Chalk one up for good coaching.

He knew how to build a team. We had a pretty diverse group in terms of talent and background, but he molded us together to believe in a system of play that required discipline and the ability to think under pressure. We had a required study hall every day before practice. That helped the marginal students like me to focus and get a start on homework and to get help from our smarter teammates. He had rules and principles that he did not compromise. When two starters were caught at a party where people were drinking, they were off the team. No questions asked. Of course that was 1963 when you could do that. Mr. Keuhl was a big reason I went into coaching and teaching.

Ironically, the other reason I went into coaching was bad coaching. My college line coach and the head coach were the antithesis of everything I thought coaching should be. Of course, their job was to win and we were never allowed to forget that. I look back on that experience and realize it was all about manipulation, domination and control. If you did something wrong in practice you ran stadium stairs in full uniform with your helmet on in 100-degree heat. Very enlightened! Our education was an afterthought.

I was a second-string center and one afternoon when practice was well into the third hour, I went to the head coach to ask if I could leave practice to make my evening class. His response was to ask me if I was there to play football or to get an education. I answered to get an education, as by now I had this figured out. I should have left then and never come back, but I persisted. The line coach preached hurting people. It was a very negative experience. I vowed after this experience that I would go into coaching and try to be the best coach I could be. I have been a bad coach at times. But when I think back on my experiences, it gets me back on track. Everyday I coach, I try to get better and make the people I work with better. What more can we ask?

Before Bo Jackson: Sam Cunningham

Sometimes as a coach you are privileged to work with an athlete. In my 37-year career I cannot say that about too many. I can with Sam Cunningham. Many of you do not even know who he is because his big days were in the 1970s as a star running back at USC, and for the Patriots in the NFL. In his football days he was known as Sam "Bam" Cunningham. Sam was the one of the first athletes I got to coach. It was my first semester coaching as a student coach at Santa Barbara High School. I was coaching the shot putters and jumpers. Sam had thrown 61'10" the previous year and was a favorite to win the state that year. He was also one of the most sought-after running backs in the nation. Sam did win the state with a throw of 64"9" mostly because of his ability and competitiveness, certainly not because anything this wet-behind-the-ears, 21-year old beginning coach had done. In the league meet Sam ran a 9.7 100-yard dash, won the 220, anchored the winning 440 relay and threw the shot over 62' at 6'3" 220 pounds!

At the track banquet Sam gave me the shot that he used to win the state meet with; (I still have it in my garage.) I had given him the shot early in the season when the shot he was using kept slipping off his hand. Afterwards he told me (in private) that the shot always weighed in overweight by three-to-four ounces, but he kept using it because it felt good in his hand. As an aside, he won the two meets leading to the state meet by a grand total of eight inches with an overweight shot put.

Sam went to USC. His freshman year we both competed in the same decathlon. This was his first and last decathlon as he focused on football after that. It was also my first decathlon. Sam scored almost 6,500 points without really having practiced four of the ten events. He did this with a 6-minute-and-20-second 1,500-meter run in flats on a dirt track because of blisters. It happened to be Bill Toomey's (the world record holder at the time) last decathlon and I remember him saying that if Sam focused on the decathlon he could someday be the world-record holder.

Beyond all of this, Sam was a great person—humble, a leader, kind and considerate, the epitome of a classy team player. His greatest fame came on a fall evening in 1970 in Birmingham, Alabama. USC was playing the University of Alabama at Legion Field. This was six years after the Civil Rights Act of 1964, but Birmingham was the bastion of the Jim Crow South. Alabama had no black players on the varsity team at the time and did everything possible to avoid playing integrated teams. Sam was not the starting fullback but he came into the game early and went on to run for 135 yards in 12 carries and score two touchdowns. This was his first varsity game.

Here is a great quote from Sam taken from the book *Turning of the Tide—How One Game Changed the South*, by Don Yaeger with Sam Cunningham and John Papadakis:

> *The thing about games is that if you go out and play really, really hard and play as well as you can and do the things you need to do, you never know when the hand of greatness is going to touch you. That night I had no clue that anything was going to happen or that anything might change because of my play. I had a great night, ran for more than 100 yards, which I only did one other time in my three years at SC. But many people have said that one evening, it changed the face of college football in the Southeastern Conference. Did I go down there trying to do that? No. I just went on a road trip trying to play. My motivation was to play well enough so that I could play the next week. That was it. It had nothing to do with changing color lines, doing anything like that. But you never know when you will get the chance to do something special.*

I was at Barnes & Noble recently, when I saw the book. I picked it up and started reading it, and when I saw the above quote, I started crying. The people sitting across from me were wondering what was wrong. Nothing was wrong, but I was crying tears of joy because I was privileged to be associated with this fine young man. Without him there might not have been a Bo Jackson.

Women in Sport

A positive trend is the continued opportunities for women to compete in sport. Unfortunately, the training and preparation of women has not kept pace with the opportunities to compete. From an endocrine (hormonal) perspective, and a socio-cultural perspective, women are different and these differences must be accounted for in training and preparation. Women are certainly more susceptible to certain injuries, specifically ACL tears; this demands that prevention programs be incorporated in daily training. To do otherwise would be remiss. There is still much misunderstanding of the role of strength training with the female athlete. Some athletes and coaches just do not recognize its importance. In many cultures it is not acceptable for women to be muscular and fit. For the female athlete to receive proper training, these barriers need to be broken down.

There is no doubt that there is a need for more qualified women in coaching. The time commitment and lifestyle serve to dissuade many women because of family obligations and the general socio-cultural attitude toward women in coaching. It was interesting to see the 2005 Women's NCAA Div. I championship game with the final two teams coached by women for the first time. Why did it take so long? Women need positive role models as coaches. They need to be mentored. The typical approach has been to take the outstanding female athlete and when she retires have her go into coaching. This approach sets them up for failure. Ability to excel in a sport seldom equates with coaching success. They need to be educated and mentored so they can truly coach. There are few women in the field of athletic development for many of the same reasons.

Where the Knee Goes

I am still amazed at the number of people who coach and teach a rule of not allowing the knee to go beyond the toes. Look at movement, watch games; if you do not progressively prepare the knee to go beyond the toes with control you are actually setting the athlete up to be hurt. Where does the knee go? It goes where it has to—as long as it goes there with *control*!

This is not a new debate. When I first started weight training in 1963, the big debate was on full squats. Were they safe? As you know, in a full squat the knee goes out over the toe. Even at that time it did not make sense to me to limit where the knee should go. Remember a full squat is breaking parallel. Even at that time, as a high school student when I did what I was taught as "strict" technique, my back hurt after squatting: we were told to do quarter squats, half squats and even bench squats (the precursor to back squats). None of them felt natural. The full squat felt right. This may have been the first time when I began to suspect that the experts did not know everything.

Around 1965 or 1966, I got hold of a book written by John Jesse. He was a pioneer in training. He was essentially a physical therapist who had a really extensive sports background. In this book, he cited a study done at the University of Texas in the 1950s where they looked at over 1,000 baseball catchers. As you know, catchers squat full and deep, and the knee goes way out over the toe. They found no unusual knee problems in that population. There was also a study published in the *Journal of Strength and Conditioning Research* in the last few years, that looked at the result of restricting forward knee movement in squatting. In essence, it said that restricting forward movement of the knee puts more stress on the low back. Remember, the body is a link system; if we restrict movement in one part, another part must make up for that movement.

Play Low Ability (PLA)

This is a concept coaches have preached for years. The ability to bend your knees and play low is crucial to success in so many sports. Kelvin Giles got me thinking about this in his presentation at the English Institute of Sports. I have now included it as a subset of my agility work. That is why we do Jim Radcliffe's Oregon sway drill. That is why we do multidirectional lunges. It must be constantly reinforced in athletes to achieve low positions in game situations. It not just about flexibility, it is also about strength and body control and awareness.

This is more than bending your knees and more drills. It demands proportional bending of ankle, knee and hip. Many young athletes today are so tight in the gastroc-soleus that they make up for it by bending more at the waist. This then sets up a cascade of negative events. They are then off balance (tipped forward). This also puts more stress on the knees.

Play Low Ability is the result of a total program that incorporates proper functional stretching, progression in movement skills that stress body awareness, and strengthening that emphasizes linkage. For hip mobility we do extensive hurdle work, dividing the hurdle work into overs and unders on different days. If they are tight in the gastroc-soleus, then we do more three-dimensional calf stretching and significantly more backward running. There is no single assessment to determine all of this but a single leg squat on a box will give a lot of good information.

Do You Believe in Magic?

That is one of my favorite songs by The Lovin' Spoonful. I do believe in magic—the magic of the body. What the body is capable of doing in movement is magical. If you take a few minutes to think about it—how we move, how we see, how we breathe, how we adapt to stress—it really is magical. To think that as coaches and therapists we can have an impact on that is quite humbling. Let's appreciate the opportunity and do it to the best of our abilities. Make it *FUNdamental* and simple— let the magic work.

Teaching Skill

This is an old paradigm I was taught early in my coaching days, to teach skill. What is neat about it, is that it encompasses all styles of learning—auditory, visual and kinesthetic:

TELL THEM—Make it brief and to the point.
SHOW THEM—Make sure you show the whole action, then the key parts, and finish with the whole action.
DO IT!—Have them do it; do the whole action at a controlled speed, then some part drills, then the whole action.

Training Camps/Preseason

I contend that more championships are lost and players wasted during the preseason than any other phase of the year. No, this is *not* the time to build and increase workload; it is the time to sharpen and fine tune with competition-appropriate training. Even testing during this time can be harmful if not carefully chosen. Endurance tests are the tests of choice, but what happens if the individual or a team tests poorly on endurance? There is no time to make any changes; if you do more work on that you will hurt them. The hay is already in the barn, as they say. The real work is done leading up to the preseason training. Remember the principle of context. The context of preseason is the final preparation for the competitive season. Competition is the goal, not training.

Aging: A Longitudinal Study

I am fascinated by aging. As I am writing this blog I am aging; as you read this blog you are aging. I have joked over the last few years that I am doing a personal aging study. I have really ramped up the study in the last month with the revival of the breakfast club. Working out with two athletes 30 years younger than me has really tested my limits. The results of the study probably will not appear in a peer-reviewed journal, but here are some preliminary conclusions:

- Aging is unforgiving and relentless.
- A good part of aging is a state of mind. If you think you are old and act old you will be older.
- Once an athlete, always an athlete, so train like one. Do not become a jogger.

- As you get older you need more recovery between hard workouts.
- Aches and pains are slow in disappearing. A niggling knee pain in your 30s will put you out of commission for several weeks in your 50s.
- Wear and tear is cumulative.
- Soreness persists.
- Often, the mind is willing, but the body is not able.
- Lifestyle and diet are even more important if you want to keep training.
- Strength training assumes more importance, both from a muscular strength perspective and from an endocrine (hormonal) perspective.
- Training is cumulative; your body does not forget. Unfortunately, it remembers the good and the bad. The old injuries are still there.

I would be very interested in other people's reactions and comments. I also recommend two books by John Jerome: *Staying With It—On Becoming An Athlete* and *On Turning Sixty-Five*. He is one of my favorite nonfiction authors. Staying With It chronicles his training as a master swimmer returning to competition in his 50s. The latter, *On Turning Sixty-Five* is, in some ways, a follow-up to see the effects 15 years later. More updates are to follow, hopefully for the next 20 or 30 years.

John Madden

Reading about John Madden's induction into the NFL Hall of Fame brought back memories of a morning in April 1967. I was a student at Fresno State College. I was also a member of the football team, a 187-pound offensive lineman, with dreams of someday coaching. In conjunction with the conclusion of spring practice there was a spring game and a clinic.

One of the speakers at the clinic was a little-known defensive line coach from San Diego State by the name of John Madden. A friend of mine had played for him at a small junior college near where I lived. He could not say enough good things about Madden. The statement that stuck with me the most was that he made football fun. When I found out he was speaking, I asked my coaches if I could attend the clinic. Needless to say it was great. He was animated, just like on TV. Chalk flying everywhere, shirt untucked. You could see and feel his passion for the game. He also talked about a simple test he used to pick his defensive linemen. It was a simple figure-eight sprint around the goal posts (two posts in those days). He said the fastest people on the test were his best players. Interesting concept, I thought. Incidentally they had a tremendous lineman that was notably undersized but very fast.

The Other 98 Percent

What does that mean? It is the 98-percent solution. I keep running into people looking for that last 2 percent. It dawned on me yesterday that most of these people had not really taken care of the first 98 percent. Instead of looking for that small edge, fully exploit the biggest part of the training puzzle. There is so much there that people overlook or just simply do not pay attention to. Pay attention to the 98 percent, fully exploit all aspects of it, and then you will see quantum leaps in performance. Little things like, consistency in the approach to training, focusing on the task at hand, living a lifestyle away from training commensurate with excellence, are all obvious things that will help to expand and exploit the 98 percent. No tricks, no shortcuts, no secrets—just good, directed training that addresses all components of athletic development.

Training to Be Hurt

Yesterday morning, we had a great training session. Unfortunately, we came back in the afternoon to begin work on acceleration mechanics. I met the athletes at a soccer and youth football complex. Big mistake! Our training was outstanding, but I could not ignore what was going on around me. It was truly amazing. I saw soccer team after soccer team start their training session with anywhere from three-to-five minutes of jogging, though really it was slogging. When they finished this waddling exercise in futility then they immediately got on the ground for stretching. They did static stretching for at least ten minutes. How do you think they felt after static stretching for ten minutes in ninety-degree heat—very lethargic and tired? That set the tempo for the practices. Amazing 15 minutes of wasted time that could have been productively used to actually warm them up and improve their athleticism. It is no wonder that we have the ACL injuries that we have in female athletes.

This scene is repeated daily everyday throughout the United States. It is not like we do not know better, but the word is not getting to those who need it most—the youth coaches. Chances are, they are parents volunteering to coach; their hearts are in the right place, but they need guidance and direction.

Connecting Links

Simplicity yields complexity. True genius lies in the ability to make the complex simple. Human movement, by its very nature, is a complex interaction of many systems. Our job as coaches and therapists is not to try to make it more complicated; anyone can do that. Look for connections and relationships. Do not get hung up on minutiae. All systems of the body work together all the time. You cannot just train the muscular system or the nervous system, or any other system in the body for that matter; they all work together to produce smooth, efficient movement.

Train and rehab the connections by using methods that promote linkage. Think of linking the ankle, knee and hip, the hip to the shoulder. This is the most effective means of staying on the "functional path" and being efficient. Training linkage transfers to efficient movement, efficient movement transfers to improved performance. How can you do this? Use movements that are multiple-plane and multiple-joint and work through the core. Think movements not muscles. Push, pull, reach, grab, extend, bend, and then combine these into bigger patterns that encourage muscle synergies. Keep it simple to be smart. Give the body credit for its innate motor genius and put it in positions to use that genius. Make it simple; make it *FUNdamental* and the complexity will follow.

Optimum Firing Patterns: Do They Exist?

Are there optimum firing patterns for various muscle groups?
According to many "experts" there are. They can put someone on a plinth and
do some manual muscle testing and tell if the hamstring is firing before the
glute or vice versa. Personally, I feel that the body is much smarter and more
adaptable than this. The body is a genius at solving whatever movement
problems are presented to it. Being a big fan of Richard Lieber, Professor of
Orthopaedics and Bioengineering at the University of California, San Diego,
I think the following quote from his excellent book, *Skeletal Muscle Structure,
Function & Plasticity—The Physiological Basis of Rehabilitation* sums it up quite
nicely:

> *The nervous system provides the signal for the muscle 'to do its thing', but
> that does not necessarily specify the details of the action. It is as if the
> nervous system acts as the central control while the muscle interprets the
> control signal into an external action by virtue of its intrinsic design.*

Roger Enoka, Ph.D., Department of Integrative Physiology at the University of
Colorado, Boulder in an even more concise statement, says: "… The function
of a muscle depends critically on the context in which it is activated."
Thinking logically, this is the way the body works; it must be adaptable just
to survive. If there were optimum or even preferred firing patterns, the body
would continually be short circuiting. As my friend, Steve Myrland, says so
eloquently: "We want bodies that are adaptable rather than simply adapted."

Progression

**Lately, I have seen progression and protocol used
interchangeably.** They are not the same. Progression is criteria-based,
and movement though a progression is based upon meeting various criteria
at each stage; this is the key. It is not a protocol, which implies set steps
that pass from one stage to the next. In progression, everyone does not
spend the same time on each step. Passage through a progression is based

on mastery of each step. Also, everyone does not have to start at the same place. It depends on the level of proficiency starting out. Let's not forget progression from year to year. You do not have to start over each year; you must build upon the previous year.

Now What?

You have done all your functional screening and you have found all these restrictions and limitations. What do you do now? How do you approach fixing those things? Can they be fixed or are they part of that individual's movement signature or fingerprint? Are these legitimate questions and concerns or am I overreacting? I know that I am a coach. As a coach my job is to produce results, do no harm and progress my athletes toward their goals. For me, the ultimate accountability is what occurs on the field. I could not help but think as I watched Roger Clemens and Greg Maddux pitch an inning last night, what would a function movement of those guys show? I think it is pretty predictable; there would be some terrific imbalances. Where do you intervene? How do you intervene? Does it matter?

Remember, everything is connected. Some connections are very visible and some are quite transparent. The body will protect where it needs to, and loosen where it needs to; it will accommodate and adapt, so let's train and rehab it as the highly adaptive organism it is. *Give the body credit for its wisdom.*

Some Lessons from the School of Life

- Know yourself—Be honest with yourself.
- Define yourself—If not, you will never be comfortable with who you are.
- Accept that change is a constant. Be a change agent.
- Lead, don't follow and don't look back to see who is following.
- Know the difference between "I can't" and "I won't."

- Never take yourself so seriously that you cannot laugh at yourself.
- Learn to listen more than you talk. That is why we have two ears and one mouth.
- Know what you know. Know what you don't know.

Weyand's Work on Running Mechanics

Someone asked me: "What is your opinion about Dr. Weyand's work?" We just had a conversation about this with Dr. Jesus Dapena, noted biomechanist from Indiana University, at the USA Track and Field Coaching School. I think the work of Dr. Weyand is sound. One of his main studies is: "Faster top running speeds are achieved with greater ground forces not more rapid leg movements", by Peter G. Weyand, Deborah B. Sternlight, Matthew J. Bellizzi, and Seth Wright, published in the *Journal of Applied Physiology*, Vol. 89, Issue 5, 1991-1999, November 2000.

I really do not see that much departure from the work of Ralph Mann. I think people are trying to make too much of the differences and are not looking closely enough at the similarities. One major difference is that Weyand's work has been mainly done on the treadmill at velocities that are slower than sprint velocities. Mann's work has been done in competition with world class athletes. To better understand sprint mechanics I think their work with the synthesis provided by Bosch and Klomp give a truer picture of what is happening at top speed. Nobody has done a good study of acceleration mechanics since Betty Atwater in the late 1970s. Unfortunately, to my knowledge, this work was never published. This is where work needs to be done.

As an aside, Dr. Weyand was a protégé of Thomas A. McMahon who did much pioneering work on track surfaces and muscle stiffness. His book is a classic work, but you better have your math and physics skills sharpened to understand it in depth. As a history major, I was able to glean some key points. By the way, McMahon was a very interesting person who tragically died in his 50s. He was also a novelist and held academic positions in several departments at Harvard University.

Magic Muscles

I call the following muscles, "the magic muscles:" gluteus medius, transverse abdominis, and internal oblique. If they can do everything people think they can do, then they must be magic! Stability is a moving target; no one muscle can be responsible for stability. It is these muscles working in synergy with other muscles that produce efficient, flowing movement that reduces and produces force effectively. As far as compensation, it does occur. There is normal and abnormal compensation. Athletes are great compensators; they know their bodies and how to efficiently accommodate. Abnormal compensation usually results from some sort of a traumatic event that forces the athlete into a position or a series of movements that they cannot handle.

Groin Injuries in Soccer

Scot Dew is a soccer coach who wrote to ask me what to do about groin injuries. First of all, do not allow the players to strike a ball until they have done a thorough warm-up. This is one of my pet peeves with soccer. They kick to warm up rather than warm up to kick. I believe that doing the mini-band series daily is important to prevent groin injuries and to warm up. In fact, it is the first thing we do in a warm-up.

Mini-Band Routine
(Band above ankles, keep tension on band at all times.)
> *Sidestep x 20 each direction*
> (Big step with lead foot, small step with following foot.)
> *Walk—Forward/Back x 20*
> (As big a step as possible.)
> *Carioca x 20*
> (Cross in front, step apart, cross behind step apart.)
> *Monster Walk—Forward/Back (wide and low) x 20*
> *Multi-plane Lunges* in strength training are very important. We also include a lunge and reach series in warm-up daily. (It probably is better

to call it a step and reach series, as the length of the lunge progresses as you get looser.)
Hurdle Walks, both over and under, are very effective prevention exercises.

Also include the following:
Crawls
(Use in warm-up and follow it with hurdle walkovers.)
Jack Knife Crawl x 5
(Walk feet to hands and then walk hands away from feet.)
Creepy Crawl x 5
(Spiderman, low and long, keep the head down.)
Tubing Leg Strength (Attach tubing low.)
(Ten reps of each exercise with each leg if before a workout. If after running do 20 reps of each leg.)
Pawing
(Essentially like a "B" Drill—Standing, face the attachment, step over the knee, emphasize out, down and pawing back.)
Hip Extension
(Standing, face the attachment, extend the leg back while keeping the leg straight.)
Adduction
(Cross the Midline—Standing, side to the attachment, keep the exercising leg in the air.)
Abduction
(Standing, side to the attachment, start with legs crossed and take the leg out—keep the exercising leg in the air.)

Prehab: A Flawed Concept

Prehab is another term that has taken on a life of its own.
There is no place for the term. Every sound training program should have an injury prevention component build into it. It should be relatively transparent. If there are intrinsic issues in a particular sport or with an individual athlete, then there should be a remedial component designed to address that. This

may seem like splitting hairs, but words create images and images create action. Remediation and injury prevention are part of a good program. I work hard to make those components transparent without de-emphasizing their importance to the athletes. The interesting thing for me is to watch these people who are putting such emphasis on prehab. They seem to have the most injuries! Could it be that the prehab is setting them up for injuries?

Remedial work is inherent in good training progressions, which goes a long way toward preventing injuries, so carefully design your progressions to incorporate a remedial component. Also, do not be in a hurry, progression takes time. The message is, remediate daily, even with elite athletes. Hide it in the warm-up and in other training tasks so they relate it to the movements of their sport.

Hamstring Injury Prevention Exercise Selection

The following is an excerpt from an article that Dean Benton and I wrote for _Sports Coach_ in Australia, Vol. 28, No. 4, "Continuum of injury prevention/performance enhancement exercise."

The placement of exercises on the continuum is ultimately determined by the relationship to the function of the hamstring in actual running. It helps to look at the continuum as progressing from a low speed, high force emphasis, to high speed/high force exercises that are ballistic in nature. At the general end of the continuum the exercises do not as closely resemble the criteria activity. As the exercises progress along the continuum, the movement pattern is similar and force time characteristics more closely resemble the actual activity. The goal of all of these is multifaceted; to improve functional strength, improve intermuscular coordination and improve the mechanics of sprinting.

GENERAL	SPECIAL	SPECIFIC
Low step-ups	Hanging horizontal bridge	Straight leg bounds
High step-up	Cable hip extension	B drills
Lunge and reach, 3 planes	Resisted moonwalks	15 degree hill sprints
Walking lunge & high knee		

Complementary Exercises:
The following training modules contain complementary exercises that should be implicit in a comprehensive strength and conditioning program. Although they may not specifically train the hamstrings they involve the hamstrings in patterns of movement that force them to work through amplitudes of movement and at speeds that prepare the hamstrings for the stresses they will encounter in sprinting and multi directional movement.

Running Technique Training
This should be fairly obvious, but the necessary attention to detail and the time required to carry this out, puts coaches off. This does not entail making the athlete conscious of hamstring firing or involvement, rather the emphasis is on the rhythm and flow of the movement. Posture and relaxation are primary considerations. This should involve work on top speed running starting at ten meters and working up to alternating periods of hitting top speed and floating at top speed.

It is also imperative to work on the mechanics of running involving curves and angles to condition the body for the differing demands that put the hamstrings at risk. Stair running is a good means to reinforce proper top speed mechanics without undo stress on the hamstrings. The stair sprints should not exceed ten seconds in duration. The emphasis is on hips over the foot at contact and tall posture.

MACH SPRINT DRILLS—the primary emphasis of these drills is to superficially strengthen the muscles used in sprinting. There is some carry-over to technique but they are primarily specific strengthening exercises. The "B" series of foreleg extension and pawing back has little relationship to technique, but it is a primary exercise to strengthen the hamstrings as they work to decelerate the foreleg. The skipping aspect of the drills serves to train the stiffness component, which is so important to learn to optimize ground contact. When executing the skips, it is imperative to actively drive the foot into the ground to set up the proper ground reaction.

LOW AMPLITUDE HOPS/JUMPS—this serves to facilitate muscle stiffness. Stiffness is the opposite of sagging, which would be the leg collapsing at ground contact. This aspect has not received as much emphasis as its role in sprinting demands. Straight leg bounds, ankle bounces and low hurdle hops all reinforce stiffness. The emphasis here should be on the knee being almost locked. Emphasize bouncing type movements, which result in very short ground contact times. Cue the athlete that the ground is hot.

HURDLE DYNAMIC HIP MOBILITY EXERCISES—It is hip mobility, or a lack thereof, that is the genesis of many hamstring problems. These drills should be incorporated daily as part of warm-up or cool-down. Without proper hip mobility the leg will not be able to work through the full range of motion. This limitation will eventually lead to flawed mechanics, especially in a fatigued state.

RESISTED HIP ABDUCTION/ADDUCTION EXERCISE—The hip abductors and adductors play a major role in stabilization. In fact, the adductor magnus is sometimes referred to as the fourth hamstring. If they are weak or not coordinated with the hamstrings more strain will be placed on the hamstrings.

FIFTEEN-DEGREE HILL SPRINTING—hill sprinting at a 15-degree grade provides an excellent means to develop good top speed mechanics. It is virtually impossible to overstride sprinting uphill.

Hamstring Strengthening

How do you strengthen the hamstring? It is necessary to understand hamstring function, in order to select effective exercises that prevent hamstring injuries and optimize sprinting performance. The nature of the injury and the phase of the stride cycle where the injury commonly occurs provides a major indication of hamstring function as well as insights into the mechanism of injury. Despite this clear evidence of hamstring function and the biarticular nature of the hamstrings, there is a continued search for ways to isolate the hamstrings in order to strengthen them. With the understanding of the eccentric role the hamstrings play in the stride cycle, some people (the authors included) searched for ways to strengthen the hamstrings eccentrically.

Unfortunately, most of those methods still relied on single joint movements, for example:
   Hamstring Curl (regardless of the position of the body).
   Ham/Glute Raise.
   Various Supine Bridging Movements.
   Kneeling Russian Hamstring Exercise.

All of the above exercises certainly do work the hamstrings eccentrically, but the problem is that they all isolate the hamstrings by working at one joint—the knee. None of the exercises contribute to intermuscular coordination nor do they work the hamstrings at anywhere near the speed necessary to transfer to performance. Furthermore, the Kneeling Russian Hamstring Exercise in particular, excessively loads the hamstring distally. All these exercises are contraindicated.

INSTRUCTION: Kneel on the ground with hands at your side. Have a partner hold firmly at your ankles. With a straight back, lean forward leading with your hips. Your knee, hip and shoulder should be in a straight line as you lean toward the ground. Do not bend at the waist. You should feel the hamstrings in the back of your thigh working. Repeat the exercise for three sets of ten, or a total of thirty reps.

Dysfunction or Functional Adaptation?

When is a dysfunction really a dysfunction? Are some of the things that people are calling dysfunctions merely adaptive responses based on their participation over time in a particular sport or activity? Is the body symmetrical, as we have been lead to believe? Is there a perfect movement pattern and technique for each activity? Do muscles really shut off? Are we hunting for things that really are not there, with the emphasis on movement dysfunction?

These are not sarcastic questions, but are really concerns based on things I have seen and heard over time. When do you train if you have these "dysfunctional" patterns? Is training bad for your health?

Active Warm-up

The warm-up is an aspect of training that is very easy to take for granted because it must be a component of each training session, and that allows it to become quite mundane. Remember, the warm-up sets the tempo for the training session. It is not separate from the workout, but an integral part of the workout. Because it is so crucial to the workout, it should be thoroughly planned to dovetail into the actual workout.

A complete and effective warm-up should be in concert with the goal of the workout. The warm-up is the transition from normal daily activity to the actual workout. It should be progressive, in that it builds in intensity in a crescendo-like manner. It must be active and dynamic, not passive and static. It is a given that the warm-up should elevate the heart rate and raise the core temperature of the muscles, but the most overlooked and perhaps the most valuable aspect of the warm-up is nervous system stimulation. The nervous system is the command and control system of the body; it must be activated. This dictates the order, selection, and tempo of the tasks that comprise the warm-up.

The warm-up consists of multiple stages that fall into two broad categories: general warm-up and specific warm-up. The stages are not equally divided; the proportion is usually 75-80 percent general to 20-25 percent specific. The stages are sequenced to work from the ground up and the core out. There is an emphasis on hip position, awareness and mobility. If there are multiple training sessions planned for a day, then each warm-up after the first should be abbreviated. The only exception to this is if there are more than six hours between workouts. Six hours seems to be the threshold when the residual effect of the previous warm-up and workout begin to diminish.

It is also important to point out that the warm-up is very individual. If the individual has a hyper and excitable makeup then often the warm-up does not have to be as long. The opposite is true for the mellow, more passive athlete. In team situations these individual considerations need to be taken into account. As the athlete progresses through their career and gains more experience, the warm-up assumes a ritual-like routine. I remember watching Edwin Moses—two-time Olympic champion in the 400-meter hurdles—warm up. His routine never varied, he did the same exercises, in the same order, no matter what the conditions. The whole routine took 45 minutes, but when he was finished he was ready to train or compete.

Competition warm-up should be different in some regards from practice warm-up. It can serve as a tool for psychological arousal or calming, as needed. Competition warm-up must be flexible to adapt to different conditions and space requirements.

For more explanation of the exercises and additional sequences see my video *Warm-up and Preparation* available at www.gambetta.com.

Please see below for a detailed program of warm-ups:

ACTIVE MULTI-STAGE WARM-UP:
   Relaxed Strides 6-8 x 50 meters at 60-70 percent

MINI BAND ROUTINE (12" BAND ABOVE ANKLES):
   1) Sidestep, 2) Walk—Forward/Back, 3) Carioca, 4) Monster Walk
BALANCE AND STABILITY:
   Single Leg Squat (Hold each position for ten counts.)
   a) Straight 2 x each leg, b) Side 2 x each leg, c) Rotation 2 x each leg

BALANCE SHIFT:
Shift and Step Right—Shift and Step Left
Forward Step Right—Forward Step Left
Back Step Right—Back Step Left

BASIC CORE (3 KG MED BALL):
Wide Rotation x 20—Walking Forward and Backward
Tight Rotation x 20—Walking Forward and Backward
Side to Side x 20—Walking Forward and Backward
Chop to Knee x 20—Walking Forward and Backward
Figure 8 x 20—Walking Forward and Backward

MULTI-DIMENSIONAL STRETCH:
Step and Reach Series (2 reps in each plane Forward/Side/Rotational)
Reach Up, Reach Out and Down, Reach Across

ACTIVE STRETCH:
Psoas, Hamstring, Adductors, Calves, Lats and Pecs as needed

CRAWLS:
Jack Knife Crawl x 5
Creepy Crawl x 5

HIP MOBILITY (FIVE HURDLES)—NOT DONE IN EVERY WARM-UP:
Hurdle Walks—Over

COORDINATION (TWO REPS OF EACH EXERCISE.):
Skip
Crossover Skip
Side Step
Carioca (low and long)
Carioca (short and quick)
Backward Run
High Knee Skip
High Knee Skip w/Rotation

More on Periodization

The following comment was sent in regard to my earlier comments on periodization.

While this certainly sounds right, I'm wondering if this comment is a research-based fact or personal impression and, if the former, the sources of it. Although I am certainly not an expert, I wonder if it perpetuates a characterization and/or stereotype of the former 'Iron Curtain' countries.

It is both research-based and personal impression-based on extensive observation, study and conversation about the training and planning methodologies of the former Eastern European countries. For example, I refer you to one of my previous posts in the archives of my blog from the *Journal of Clinical Chemistry*. Read the work of Franke and Berendok; without extensive doping support, the East German sport machine would have been a shadow of what it was. I am not sure what you mean by the stereotype of the former Eastern European countries. I try to stay away from stereotypes, but for those countries, sport was part of national policy. Success in sport was closely tied to the Communist ideology. One only has to read their coaching manuals and see the opening chapters on Marxist-Leninist dialectics. This is not meant to denigrate the progress and innovations they made in sport, but we must always put their writing in the context of the social/cultural milieu that existed at the time.

Periodization is a concept not a model. Unfortunately, over the years it has been portrayed as a strict model, but it is not. As a concept, periodization is an educated attempt to predict future performance based on evaluation of previous competition and training results. It brings the future into the present so that we can do something about it. It is achieved through planning and organization of training into a cyclical structure to develop all global motor qualities in a systematic, sequential and progressive manner for optimum development of the individual's performance capabilities. We need to get away from the traditional focus on the models of periodization that were developed and refined in Socialist/Communist societies that had strict control over every aspect of the athletes' lives, including systematic doping.

That is not our sporting culture. The focus should shift to the process of adaptation and the underlying concepts to achieve optimum adaptation by applying a systems approach to planning training. This implies that everything must fit into the context of a larger whole. A system is an integrated whole. Changing one part of the system changes the whole system. Everything is interconnected. The elements of the system are only viable because of the relationship between the parts.

Planning is essential to sport performance regardless of the level of competition. The traditional focus has been on the long-term plan. It has been my experience that the longer the period of time for the plan, the less applicable the plan will be. To be more effective, the long-term planning should focus on global themes and training priorities based on competition performance, training and testing data from previous years. The detailed planning of the microcycle and the individual training sessions is where focus needs to be for planning to be more effective and practical.

There are contemporary issues that necessitate re-evaluation of the traditional concepts of periodization:

1. There is a serious decline of basic physical fitness levels and fundamental movement skills at the developmental level. Even elite athletes do not have the broad base of movement skills that the athletes had when I began coaching in the late '60s. This necessitates a remedial emphasis throughout the athlete's career because this was not incorporated in a foundation.

2. The reality of the extended competitive schedule that exists today is quite demanding. In classical periodization, competition was strictly controlled. This is not a reality today. It is not unusual for a professional soccer player to play 70 matches in a season. At the youth level, it is the norm for a baseball player to play 100 games in a year. This reality forces a revision of the classical ideas of periodization. This competitive schedule will not change so we must adapt our planning to this reality.

3. In traditional periodization models, developed in the former Eastern-bloc nations, there was a drug influence/bias. The revelations from the former GDR (German Democratic Republic) exposed that the reality of their planning was the cyclical application of systematic doping. This has a profound effect on the frequency and intensity of training and, most importantly, on the ability to recover. To base training methodologies on information derived from this system is fundamentally flawed, yet this is what has been done and is continued today. The majority of the traditional literature on periodization has been written by people who were part of this system. We must take this into account in planning for our system which does not have the strict control of the former Eastern-bloc nations.

4. There has been an overemphasis on volume-loading relating to the previous point. Systematic doping enables the athlete to tolerate significantly higher work loads. The published programs from the former Eastern European countries always emphasized the periodic increase of tons lifted, meters run, etc., linked to incremental performance improvement from year to year. It turns out that the volume loading increases in those programs were closely linked to changes in dosages of anabolic substances. For the non-drugged athlete, volume has to be increased gradually, and in many sports it should not be the primary emphasis.

5. We must apply the improved understanding of the human adaptive response to various training stimuli, especially in terms of neural and endocrine (hormonal) system response. From current research our knowledge of the adaptive response has increased significantly. This needs to be applied in order to devise more exact training plans based on what we know of the science of adaptation.

Spectrum Approach

The dictionary defines *spectrum* as a broad range of related values or qualities, ideas or activities. The spectrum approach is the cornerstone of Functional Training and Rehab as I define it. Training consists of a movement across a spectrum of activities and training methods. You do not stay in one place. It is not segmented, but a blending of one method into another. At different times of the year and in a career, the emphasis will be on different points on the spectrum.

As an example, look at the strength training spectrum. It begins with body weight and progresses to high force, slower speed lifting, which in turn progresses to high speed, high force ballistic work. Depending on the sport and individual needs, it is entirely possible for one athlete to stay on one point on the spectrum for a relatively long period of time. This is not an arbitrary decision but criteria- and need-based. It is essential to have a method to determine where you need to be on the spectrum. This should be evidence- and testing-based.

What is Functional Training?

This is something I am continually asked about. I must admit I have struggled to give a good answer, but based on all of my reading, and some discussions I've had with like-minded professionals in England, I am going to make an attempt at defining functional training.

I am not sure it can be strictly defined because it encompasses such a broad area. First, we must define function. The definition I use is that it is integrated, multidirectional movement. Everything we do as long as we are alive is functional, but it is really a matter of how functional, relative to what we are preparing for. One of the dictionary definitions of function is, "A thing depends and varies with something else." It does not mean that you don't lift weights. It does mean that you are acutely aware of context and the interrelationship of physical qualities and systems of the body.

Functional training incorporates a full spectrum of training designed to elicit the optimum adaptive response appropriate for the sport or activity being trained for. It incorporates a kaleidoscope of methods systematically applied to improve all systems of the body. No one system is emphasized to the exclusion of another. No one method or physical quality becomes an end unto itself. Each athlete is a case study of one. Each athlete brings something different to the table. It is characterized by integration of movement and a spectrum approach. By spectrum approach, I mean moving along a spectrum of methods and activities relevant to the method being utilized. At best, I can tell you that this definition of functional training is not new. It is something that has characterized good training and rehab programs for a long time.

Core Training

Effective and functional core training is based on two simple principles: Train core strength before extremity strength. A strong, stable core will allow the extremities to better do their job; therefore, we should train the core first in a training session and in a training program.

Dynamic postural alignment is the foundation for training. Posture and a strong and stable core are integrally related. Posture is a dynamic quality. The larger core muscles known as *anti-gravity muscles* play a major role in maintaining a sound, functional athletic posture. We need to shift our thinking away from posture as a still picture or a posed position. Posture must be assessed relative to the athlete's event. Each sport has its own specific posture and each individual within the sports has his or her own posture. The combination of the two allows for much variability. Our goal should not be to fit everyone into certain parameters, rather it should be to understand what each athlete brings to their event and adjust accordingly.

An important assumption is that the body is fundamentally asymmetrical. It is unrealistic to think of muscular balance right to left or front to back. We must think of proportionality. The core muscles play a major role in dynamic posture because the large muscles of the core act as anti-gravity muscles that give the body structural integrity. This allows the limbs to position and reposition according to the demands of the activity.

Balance is a key aspect of movement that is closely related to the core. Balance is a dynamic quality because movement is dynamic. Balance is control of one's center of gravity, control of body angles and unstable equilibrium. Movement is a state of dynamic equilibrium consisting of a constant interplay of imbalance and balance, with the body constantly trying to regain balance to perform efficient movement. There is a continual reaction to gravity and external forces such as the playing surface, the opponent, etc. The muscles of the core play a decisive role in balance because of the location and function of the core muscles; therefore, core training and balance training are synonymous.

The core is an integrated functional unit consisting of the lumbo-pelvic-hip complex, the thoracic and cervical spine. It is a muscular corset that lends integrity and support to the body. The core is the center of the body, the thickest part of the body. The core is where all movement is modulated. It is more than six-pack abs. The core works as an integrated functional unit that accelerates, decelerates, and dynamically stabilizes the body during movement. All movement is relayed through the core. The core is a swivel joint between the hips and the shoulders, which: 1) allows the entire body to accelerate the limbs, 2) allows the entire body to decelerate the limbs, and 3) allows the entire body to support a limb.

Core Strength Assessment

The traditional method of assessment is isolated, and is usually in a prone or supine position seeking to isolate strength of individual muscles. The functional assessment is integrated and movement-oriented in a standing position, or a position that simulates the posture of the sport. A simple, qualitative analysis consists of simply taking video of the athlete doing their respective sport activity from the front, side and rear if possible, and judging the quality of the movement. Also, take a video of a typical training activity and judge the quality of the movement. Look for patterns, similarities and differences. Quantitative assessment has two components:

Assessment Driven from the Top Down
Medicine Ball Chest Pass
      Off Two Legs
      Off One Leg
Medicine Ball Overhead Throw
      Off Two Legs
      Off One Leg
Medicine Ball Rotational Throw
Compare distance right and left

Assessment Driven from the Bottom Up
Balance Tests
Excursion Tests
Lunge, Jump, Hop Tests

After the core strength assessment program to design a core training program, select the exercises carefully by considering all of the following:

- Demands of the sport.
- Demands of the event or position.
- Physical qualities of the athlete.
- Dynamic postural analysis.
- Injury history.
- Performance and training history.

As in any good training program progression is the key. It is essential to achieve mastery of each step before moving to the next step. Start with easy and simple basic movements and progress to harder and more complex movements. I have found it more effective to emphasize a few, simple, basic movements and then add variations off of those movements, rather than adding more exercises. Therefore, the foundation of an effective core training program is a few exercises mastered and done well. Choose exercises that work the core in all planes of motion:

- Trunk Flexion and Extension (Sagittal plane).

- Lateral Flexion (Frontal plane).
- Trunk Rotation (Transverse plane).
- Combinations (Tri-plane).
- Catching (Dynamic stabilization in all three planes).

Planned Performance Training

Planned Performance Training is a term I like to use instead of periodization. I think it is more descriptive of the whole process. The other day I was talking to someone about what classically is called periodization, and it made me realize that in this country, we just don't get it. Yes, it is about time and planning, but more importantly it is about timing of the application of the appropriate training stimulus. When you do what you do is the key. In order to have an effective plan and make it work you must know where you are at all times. This requires constant monitoring of training.

The Zombie Mode

I just finished reading an interesting book, *The Three Pound Enigma—The Human Brain and the Quest to Unlock Its Mysteries*, by Shannon Moffett. In the chapter called, "Mining the Brain" she interviews Dr. Christof Koch and Francis Crick. Crick is famous for his work with James Watson on the discovery of the helical structure of DNA. Basically, he devoted much of the remainder of his career to the study of brain function. How does this all relate to movement and coaching? Well, over the past several years I have been convinced that to better understand movement and train movement we need to better understand brain function. There has been an explosion of research in this area. Much of it is way too complex for an old coach like me to understand. But at times I am able to cull bits and pieces from my exploration.

It was late at night when I was reading this book. As I was dozing off, this concept jumped off the page at me. The concept is that of the zombie mode. Koch and Crick have determined that most of what happens in the brain occurs at an unconscious level. In scientific terminology these are called cortical reflexes but the authors have termed them the zombie mode. What appealed to me about this concept is the fact that I have heard some of the great coaches who I know (who were not into brain research) in essence, say the same thing. One coach I know calls it pushing the button. You push one button and it turns on a cascade of movement. Koch and Crick point out that the zombie reflex is faster than our conscious mind. They use the example of tennis:

> If you play tennis well, most of it is totally at the zombie level. The ball approaches at high speed and your body executes the right sequence of motion to intercept the ball with your racket and return it. There is almost no delay between sensing the ball and reacting to it. It's all smooth motion, egoless, thoughtless.

They point out that a combination of the zombie reflex and slower stereotyped responses are what enable us to run complex movement schema.

It seems that our goal as professionals working with movement is to first, recognize this phenomenon and second, to put the body in positions to activate this phenomenon. In my opinion, the foundation for these actions is developed early. That is why we need to get moving, allow kids to explore movement and test their limits. Food for thought.

Becoming an Athletic Development Professional

I have been contacted by several people who asked me to write what it takes to be an athletic development professional, as they are looking to get into the field:

PASSION—A genuine enthusiasm for what you do. Not just when there are crowds and on game day, but everyday.

EXPERIENCE—Train for, and coach, several sports. There is no substitute for having to put yourself on the line on game day as a player or a coach. This is essential. This does not mean you have to be a star, but at least participate.

STUDY AND OBSERVE—Get around great coaches. See how they work. See how they praise and scold. Learn everything they do. I once followed a German track coach, Gerd Osenberg, around for a week. I wrote down everything he did. I used to go to the 49ers training camp in the early '70s because they had a good linebacker coach. I still use some of those drills today.

LEARN AND RESEARCH—Read scientific, coaching, and technical journals. Get away from the Internet and go for straight facts. Study video.

PRACTICE—Get proficient at the skills you must teach. Be able to capably demonstrate the movements. Know skill progressions and how to teach.

BE ORGANIZED—Plan and have a contingency plan. Be on time and stay late.

LOOK THE PART—Get fit, dress the part and dress appropriately.

COMMUNICATION SKILLS—Sharpen them. Realize all the dimensions of communication.

HAVE A LIFE—Take care of your family and reserve some time for yourself.

As a last thought, remember it takes at least 20 years to be an overnight success.

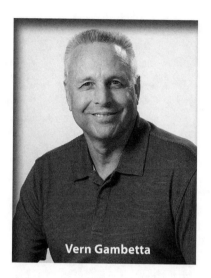

Vern Gambetta

Vern is Director of Gambetta Sports Training Systems. He is considered a pioneer of functional sports training. Vern's coaching experience spans over 40 years at all levels of competition in a variety of sports. His coaching background is rooted in track and field. He is a popular speaker and writer on conditioning topics, having lectured and conducted clinics throughout the world. He has authored over 100 articles and seven books on various aspects of training. He received his BA from Fresno State University and his teaching credential with a coaching minor from University of California Santa Barbara. Vern attended Stanford University and obtained his MA in Education with an emphasis in physical education.

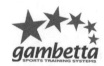

www.gambetta.com • www.functionalpathtraining.typepad.com